D0891285

Dr. Bryant Stamford's
WEIGHT LOSS READER

*Sane Strategies For Losing Body Fat and
Keeping It Off Without Crash Diets*

Dr. Bryant Stamford's

WEIGHT LOSS
READER

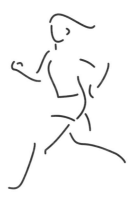

*Sane Strategies For Losing Body Fat
and Keeping It Off Without Crash Diets*

BIOSYNERGIC
HEALTH PRESS

To my countless mentors who have taught me that love is more powerful than fear; that being myself is the best me I can be; that true success is having enough; that unorthodox thinking is OK; and that common sense is a rare commodity that is worth cultivating.

Published by:
Biosynergic Health Press
407 Lake Pointe Trace
Louisville, KY 40245

ISBN 0-9714337-0-4

Printed in the United States of America

ACKNOWLEDGMENTS

I would like to thank and acknowledge the Louisville *Courier-Journal* for allowing me the privilege of writing my column, The Body Shop, for the past 25 years. The visibility afforded me in the newspaper has allowed me to teach and advise tens of thousands of readers and has attracted affiliations and experiences that otherwise would not have been possible. I am thankful that I have been given permission to reproduce some materials from The Body Shop in this book. Thanks also to *Physician & Sportsmedicine* and *Kentuckiana HealthFitness* for allowing me to reproduce some written materials.

I thank and acknowledge the University of Louisville, a respected center of higher learning, for nurturing my growth and development, for promoting my professional efforts, for allowing me freedom of expression, and for giving me the opportunity to meet and learn from many great and talented people. I am grateful for my many students who have taught me much over the years, including the value and rewards gleaned from finding unique and tender individuals hidden beneath confident and well-crafted exteriors.

I am grateful to the many individuals who have faith in my guidance and who have been willing to share their journey with me. Among these are many courageous women who wage a ferocious battle against the odds in everyday life, but are never beaten down. Their stories are reflected throughout this book.

CONTENTS

PART II — FOR WOMEN (and for those who care about them)

PREFACE

I have been writing about diet, health and exercise issues for more than 25 years. I'm not the smartest guy in the world, so, in order for me to make sense out of things, I have to break them down into simple terms that I can easily understand. This has molded my style of taking "rocket science stuff" and presenting it in "everyday" words. This seems to be what many folks appreciate most about my books and columns, and I have endeavored to sustain that approach throughout this book.

This is a collective work, spanning many years of writings from my newspaper column, The Body Shop, which appears weekly in Louisville's *The Courier-Journal*, and is syndicated by Gannett. I also have written for a number of other publications over the years, and some of these writings are included as well.

Although I have borrowed from my columns and experiences in preparing this book, I must emphasize that this book is much more than a collection. I have selected items that represent my current philosophy and are, in my opinion, the most valuable and usable to readers. I have organized them to flow seamlessly and logically, as one would expect from a book viewed as a teaching tool and reference. I have updated and added new materials to fill in gaps and make the information comprehensive and applicable.

With that said, please note: This book is not intended to be encyclopedic in scope—the economics of the publishing world won't allow that. Instead, it was necessary for me to choose one major area of concentration, and I have selected the topic that seems to be of most concern to the largest number of people—

body weight and weight management. Future volumes will cover exercise and fitness, strength and muscle building, preventive health, heart disease, healthy nutrition, alternative/ complementary medicine, successful aging, beating stress, and other issues.

Until recently, my Body Shop column was structured in a question-and-answer format. I will include some of those questions from readers, and my responses, in this book to expand a point or introduce another slant on the issue at hand. To protect confidentiality and broaden interest, I have rewritten the letters, often combining aspects of several letters into one.

I ask that those of you who are professionals forgive my taking license at times for the purpose of communicating most easily and effectively with a lay audience. My use of the word "calorie" for example, is used because of its familiarity, rather than the correct term, "kilocalorie", which often is confusing to lay readers.

If you are not familiar with my writings, I must warn you that my philosophy at times surprises readers and seems unusual, if not downright contrary, offbeat and strange. Letters, e-mails, and calls from readers have characterized my writing as anything from absurd to refreshing, from revolting to inspiring. Thankfully, the vast majority of responses are overwhelmingly positive, and for that I am grateful.

A keystone element of my philosophy is my belief in people and their ability to grow and change. And I believe the first step toward growth and change is real knowledge about what's going on.

Thus, this book was lovingly crafted as a first step toward meaningful change.

This book comprises two parts. The first part is an overview and a common-sense approach to losing weight and keeping it off. It contains everything you need to know to win the battle of the bulge. But this is not a diet book with recipes and so on. I've already written such a book; it's called *The Jack Sprat Low-fat Diet: A 28-day Heart-Healthy Plan You Can follow the Rest of Your Life.* "Jack Sprat" provides details on exactly how to eat from day to day to be successful, and it's loaded with tasty recipes. After reading this book, you will have a strong background and will be ready to take on the specifics of a sound diet plan like that in "Jack Sprat." (See Part I, # 6 for an overview of the Jack Sprat low-fat diet.)

The second part of this book is devoted to weight management issues that are of particular concern to women. Men will benefit from reading this section, too, by developing an appreciation for some of the unfair burdens our society places on women. Issues covered include an examination of realistic versus fantasized expectations of what the female figure should be, and how women can liberate themselves from the tyranny of the too-thin, cover-girl look which dominates the American scene.

I hope you enjoy this book as much as I enjoyed putting it together. More important, it is my wish that you take something away from it which enhances your quality of life and your happiness. Take care, God bless, and read on.

* Many of the materials reprinted by permission are owned and copyrighted by *The Courier-Journal*, *Physician & Sportsmedicine*, and *Kentuckiana HealthFitness*.

PART I

WATCHING YOUR WEIGHT

INTRODUCTION

I f we define overweight as being at least 20 percent above a desirable weight, we see that more and more Americans are entering the corpulent ranks each year. In 1980, 26 percent of us were considered overweight. A decade later, the percentage was up to 34 percent. Add another decade, and today we find that more than half of us qualify. Amazing!

Why are we getting fatter? We are, by and large, an inactive society, with small pockets of highly active individuals who run marathons and ride mountain bikes. The most sedentary among us, the bottom 25 percent, have not budged from the couch in the last decade. These people staunchly avoid exercise and gain weight progressively as they age. Unfortunately, over the past ten years not much headway has been made in bolstering the ranks of those who regularly engage in moderate activity (up two percent), and vigorous activity (up 1 percent).

How are we Americans doing with our diets? Dietary fat consumption is down two percent in the past decade. Hooray! Unfortunately, this two percent drop is misleading, because caloric intake is up, and most of this increase is from sugar, which contributes to obesity and creates its own set of problems.

With all the bad press on obesity, the obvious health implications (diabetes, hypertension, etc.) and the ruinous effects on self esteem, why can't we call a halt to the process that creates obesity? For starters, changing a habit is difficult, and eating habits may be the most ingrained of all. A forty year-old has a forty year habit to contend with. That's tough, but it's more complicated than that.

Americans aren't much good when it comes to long range thinking and planning, and we certainly don't do well in preventing problems. On the contrary, our strength is our ability to rise to the occasion, to rally the troops in a crisis. When we get motivated to act, we go all-out, taking on too much too soon, fighting all the dragons at one time. This approach can serve us well on some battlefields, but in the battle of the bulge, it's a disaster. As a rule of thumb, the greater the change you attempt, the more likely you are to fail. Put another way—when it comes to weight control, zeal is a no-no that will do you in, because the faster the weight comes off, the faster it returns. I discuss this in great detail in several articles, especially numbers 1 through 4.

Americans also are pampered, spoiled and lazy. We believe we can live any way we like without negative consequences. We want gas guzzler cars, but cry foul when oil supplies run short and prices at the pump skyrocket. We want to eat whatever we want, but feel abused and victimized when we grow fat and unhealthy. But instead of making meaningful changes to rectify the situation, we sit back and wait for science to bail us out.

Science feeds this thirst for "cures," bombarding us with information about medical breakthroughs that will save us from ourselves. Discovery of the "fat gene" was supposed to lead to therapies that would solve the obesity problem. Fake fat and fake sugar were supposed to rescue us from our own taste buds. Miracle meds like fen-phen were supposed to knock out our appetite and help us melt the weight off painlessly. Such developments encourage us to do nothing for ourselves.

Another problem is our access to information, and misinformation. The low-fat diet was once thought to be the answer, but it's under attack, and high-fat diets are now high profile. How can a high-fat diet be healthy? What gives? There are no easy answers to such questions, but there *are* answers. And once you read this book and understand the issues, you'll know what went wrong with most low-fat diets, and why a high-fat diet is a bad alternative. You'll also learn the best fat-fighting strategies.

The only realistic approach to weight control is to limit your attack. Focus your attention on one small item at time and proceed gently and slowly. I suggest starting your attack by learning as much as you can about the enemy. Read on.

1. WHY DIETS DON'T WORK

This year millions of Americans will set out on a crusade to lose weight. Most have gone on many similar crusades in years past, and each time they have failed. But, despite repeated failures, they are convinced this one will be different. This one has a glitzy new title which promises quick weight loss that is easy, comfortable and sustainable. This one is the "Mega-Galactic, Turbo-Charged, Instant-Weight-Be-Gone Diet" that is sweeping Las Vegas and Beverly Hills, knocking pounds off the rich and famous. This one has an honest to goodness medical doctor who peers out at you from a book jacket or the TV screen, touting the benefits to be derived from secret food combinations that no one ever thought about before — combinations that allow you to eat anything your heart desires, from cheesecake to French fries to prime rib, and still lose weight. Better yet, you don't have to eat tasteless vegetables, legumes, fiber and whole grains.

Will it work? Of course it will. The authors and publisher give their solemn promise. Of the million people who buy the book, many will have the gumption to stick with the diet for months, and in the process they will lose a bunch of weight. Success? Seemingly so. But wait, let's look into the future. The weight that was lost comes back, and brings some buddies along with it. But what about those with great resolve who stick it out longer. Wow! Their weight loss is tremendous. And so is the backlash that inevitably occurs when they dump the diet.

You'd think we Americans would someday have a "duh" experience when it comes to the notion of dieting. Our society is getting fatter year by year, and yet more people are dieting, with as many as two-thirds of adults trying to lose weight. Doesn't add up, does it? You'd think we'd stop to realize that if any of the hundreds of sure-fire diets that have come and gone in the last 30 years really worked, there would be no need for new diets. There would be one bona fide approach that truly works, and everyone who is interested in losing weight and keeping it off would go there for guidance and help. Instead, we keep reaching, time and again, for the magic bullet. Comic Totie Fields said it best: "I've been on a diet two weeks, and all I've lost is two weeks!"

Here's a news flash. The only diet plan that works, that can work, is the one that lasts the rest of your life. It's not a diet, in other words, at least not a diet in the sense that we've all come to accept. Only through long-range lifestyle changes can one lose body fat and keep it off. Simply put, you must invest the same type of effort that brought on those unwanted pounds in the first place. You must reverse the process.

A good analogy: You're out hiking in the woods and after several hours you realize you are lost. What would you do? Obviously, as best you could, you would retrace your steps. You also would realize you had invested hours of effort already and had come a long way and that you'd better pace yourself on the way back so as not to fatigue and run out of gas. Common sense would dictate that, as stated above, you reverse the process. Obviously, you wouldn't sprint off in a different direction, hoping that by some miracle it might bring you back quickly to civilization. The voice of common sense inside would warn you not to do this, because it would only cause you to become more lost and less likely to make it home safely.

If this analogy makes sense to you when it comes to hiking, it should make sense to you when it comes to dieting. Americans are lost in our obesity, and in an attempt to find our way out of this dilemma we sprint. But we sprint without knowing where we are going or why, and in the process we become more lost than ever. Know this: every sprint leads nowhere except to exhaustion, and every short cut is a farce, a waste of time and effort ultimately causing you to become fatter as a result. Every quick solution leads to the up and down pattern called yo-yo dieting, which has become a way of life in this country.

Survival of the fattest?

Americans are too fat, and we're getting fatter all the time. That's not news — we all know that. And we know the reasons. Too much fat in the diet. Too many calories. Not enough fruits and vegetables. Not enough fiber. Too much TV. Not enough exercise. The list goes on. While these are obvious contributors, there are other forces operating which need to be addressed if we are to fully understand the nature of the enemy we face. Two of these forces are: (1) our natural desire and remarkable ability to store body fat; and (2) the subtle nature of the fat storage process which escapes our attention until we are captured. Let me explain.

According to Charles Darwin, the fittest survived. The fittest were the best hunters, the fiercest warriors, the most productive and dominant members of primitive society. Indeed, being fit, fast, and strong was a huge advantage back then. But being the fittest didn't always translate into the best odds of survival. The reason is, being fit generally means being lean, and being lean doesn't help much when you are in the middle of a famine with nothing to eat. On the contrary, having an ample storehouse of energy to carry you through times when food was scarce probably meant the difference between living and dying.

So, who survived? Obviously, it was those who were best at carrying around stored energy in the form of body fat. The survivors were those with a sluggish metabolism; those with the ability to efficiently convert dietary fat and carbohydrates to body fat; those with a powerful, turbo-charged pancreas capable of pumping out mega-doses of insulin at the drop of a hat; and those with a propensity toward creating new and hungry fat (adipose) cells for greater fat storage capacity. And after the famine, when the survivors, Chubby Chet, the cave man, and Corpulent Corrine, the cave woman, met and fell in love and he dragged her off to his cave, the result was offspring — our ancestors — blessed with an outstanding ability to store fat. This blessing has, of course, become a curse in our modern society where food is plentiful and there is a fast food restaurant on every corner eager to push greasy, fatty foods in our face.

The problem of too much body fatness seems obvious, doesn't it? It is, at least to the outside observer. All you have to do is visit the nearest shopping mall, prop yourself on a bench and watch passers by. What do you see? Pot bellies, love handles, bulging hips, thighs and butts. Fatness is blatantly abundant. But to each of us as individuals, looking at the problem from within our own bodies, the situation is far from obvious. In fact, the problem is so subtle it invariably catches us by surprise, and by then, the problem is so large it requires major lifestyle changes, if not a complete overhaul.

How can a bulging belly be subtle? How can it sneak up on us? It's easy. That belly didn't appear overnight. In fact, if you are a typical American, it accumulated over many years, one small bit at a time. It's the residual from the fat gain that occurs annually when the weather turns sour, the days get shorter, and the Thanksgiving-to-New Year's holiday season begins. This deadly trio packs on the pounds, then we spend the rest of the year taking it off. And we do, except for a hardly noticeable pound or two of fat. This gradual accumulation over many years is called creeping obesity.

We men leave high school in size 28 jeans. In college we advance to size 30, then by graduation to 32. Our first real job (a job with career potential and benefits) boosts us to 34. Marriage pumps us to 36, and a total lack of physical activity thereafter ensures a 38 and a gradual trudge to a 40. But the transition is gradual and all the while our blossoming fatness escapes our attention. That's not to say we are completely ignorant of what's going on. Rather, we rationalize and avoid as long as possible having to come to grips with our situation.

But one day, as our waistline continues to expand, we inevitably are forced to confront reality. The scene may play out something like this. My stomach is churning and growling and it's keeping me awake. I toss and turn in the middle of the night until, full of frustration, I stumble into the bathroom seeking relief in the medicine cabinet. Because my mind is preoccupied and I'm not thinking clearly, I violate one of my most guarded principles. I turn on the light and confront my naked self in front of a full length mirror. YIKES! Is that ME? I'm FAT! My reaction is as if the Fat Fairy (the Tooth Fairy's cousin) visited last night and left me with an additional 30 pounds of fat around my waist.

Another scenario is the upcoming high school reunion or the wedding of one of our children. Contemplation of such events causes critical self examination, seeing ourselves as we really are, and admitting that, yes, we are too fat. It's time for a change. It's time to reduce. In desperation, we reach for the nearest, quickest fix — the crash diet. And in so doing, we sow the seeds of our own destruction, guaranteeing failure regardless of our intentions and the degree of effort applied.

Formula for failure

How will you know the diet you have selected is nothing more than a fool's errand? It's easy. Every failed diet that comes along has a core of characteristics which ensures failure.

First is the promise of rapid weight loss. This one is tricky, because some diets do effect quick weight loss. But it was your intention to lose unsightly and health destroying *body fat*, not *muscle*. Unfortunately, rapid weight loss can only be taken from your muscles. There are many reasons for this, but simply put, when you challenge your body by going on a crazy diet, it clings to your fat stores like a security blanket.

Is this logical? You bet. Look at it from your body's point of view. If I am my body and I perceive you are trying to starve me to death, who is my best friend? The answer is, the fat I have stored. It will keep me alive while I undergo this period of starvation, and I will want to use it sparingly to provide fuel and make it last as long as possible.

If I'm clinging to my body fat, and still losing weight rapidly, I must be losing muscle. Herein lies the key to failure. If fat is my friend while on the diet, muscle is my enemy. Muscle is high maintenance tissue which gobbles up energy. Get rid of muscle and you lower your metabolism, reducing the difference between the limited supply of calories you take in on the diet versus the number you expend. The more favorable the balance, the better your chances for survival. This is a wise decision as far as the body is concerned, but it undermines all efforts to lose weight by severely cutting calories.

Muscles are created to be easy targets for sacrifice when the going gets rough. They are mostly water and yield only about 700 usable calories (kcals) per pound. This is why you can drop many pounds of muscle quickly. By comparison, one pound of fat supplies 3500 calories, and thus you can drop five pounds of muscle in the time it would take to drop only one pound of fat.

This is why every crash diet guarantees quick weight loss, and why some work. It's also why everyone is so excited in the early stages of one of these diets. The pounds seem to melt off effortlessly, and, basically, they do. Losing muscle mass is as easy as staying in a hospital bed for a week or casting a broken limb. Neither requires the least bit of effort, yet each will result in the quick loss of pounds of muscle. For all intents and purposes you seem to be getting something for nothing. But do you ever get something that is worthwhile for nothing? Of course not.

The tortoise and the hare

The tortoise always beats the hare, because the tortoise paces itself for the long haul, whereas the hare burns out quickly. Here are some things to consider that will help you avoid the pitfalls of the hare, and be successful like the tortoise.

1. Jump on the tortoise bandwagon and aim to lose weight *slowly*. Lose no more than 1 pound per week. You can lose more, up to 2 pounds per week, if you exercise vigorously an hour or more daily. Lose at a faster rate, and you'll know you have hooked up with the hare and are losing muscle, not fat. (For more on this, see Chapter 2.)

2. Beware of approaches that are negative and emphasize deprivation, bordering on starvation. Depending on your size, men need at least 1500-1800 calories per day, and women need 1200-1400. Ironically, without an adequate daily caloric intake, your body will have trouble burning off fat. Besides being unhealthy and self-defeating, a semi-starvation diet requires unrealistic will power and cannot last long.

3. As a rule of thumb, the greater the change you attempt the less likely you are to stick with it. So, make changes gradually and in small increments. It takes about 30 days to begin to establish a habit, so take a small piece of the puzzle, master it completely, then add another piece.

4. Stay away from extreme measures, like cutting out carbohydrates, or eating only foods from select food groups. Your body needs variety to function well and be healthy.

5. Be gentle on yourself and allow yourself a sizeable margin of error. There will be days when you don't feel like following the rules. Fine. Fall off the wagon for a day or two, then get back on. Because you are making lifestyle changes that are ongoing, falling off here and there is natural, and represents a mere blip on the scale. This differs from crazy crash diets which allow no margin of error — fall off the wagon, and the diet is over.

6. Set flexible and realistic goals. Believe it or not, losing as little as 10 pounds of body fat can make a sizeable difference in your appearance and your health. (Note the emphasis on losing body fat and not body weight!) Accomplishing this loss of 10 pounds over a three month period would seem like a pretty easy goal, and it is. But it's also beneficial and productive.

7. You need a comprehensive approach, which includes exercise. Although food intake is probably 80 percent of the battle, you will never be ultimately successful without a generous amount of physical activity added to the mix. This doesn't mean you have to huff and puff and sweat bullets. But it does mean you have to be consistent, doing something that moves your body for a prolonged period of time on a daily basis. Walking fits the bill perfectly.

8. Just as you would in other areas of your life, apply some common sense. Eating a piece of grapefruit won't cancel all the fat and calories from eating a huge piece of chocolate cake. If it seems too good to be true, it is.

The bottom line

There's an old saying: "You can't cheat an honest man." If you apply a little honesty to your weight management efforts and quit searching for the magic bullet, you won't be victimized by flim-flamming diet entrepreneurs out to make a quick buck on your naivete. Good luck and go slow.

The cabbage soup diet

The cabbage soup diet is the perfect example of a hot new diet that sweeps the country, then is gone. What's different about the cabbage soup diet is that it seems to cycle in and out, disappearing for a number of years, then, like the proverbial bad penny, reappearing from out of the blue. This diet is touted as coming from a hospital diet plan used to prepare patients for surgery, but no hospital will claim responsibility for it. Moreover, it has been universally condemned by nutritionists and dietitians.

Even so, recently it was incredibly popular and in demand, and hospitals all over the country were being besieged by calls asking about it. The cabbage soup diet and other similar approaches are seductive because of their rapid weight loss and quick-cure claims. In fact, in all my years of watching the diet landscape, the cabbage soup diet has produced the quickest and largest weight losses I have ever witnessed or heard of, reaching as much as 11 pounds in one week! Based on what you now know about crash diets, this seems pretty crazy, doesn't it? Sure, but even so, at any given time millions of Americans are following similar diets, because of all the reasons cited above. And because of all the reasons one should not subscribe to such a foolish approach to weight loss, less than a fraction of 1% of the millions who follow such diets will lose weight and keep it off for a year or more. Your body won't tolerate losing muscle and water for long.

The cabbage soup used in the diet contains green onions, green peppers, scallions, tomatoes, celery, cabbage, V-8 juice, onion soup mix, and beef bouillon. There is nothing magical in these ingredients. You lose weight fast because you are starving yourself. Let's take a closer look.

The cabbage soup diet is a seven day plan which virtually starves your body for the first four days. You eat soup which is not unhealthy (except for the high salt content), but it doesn't come close to satisfying your body's nutritional needs. Over the first four days of the diet, you depend on the soup as the backbone, plus fruits, vegetables, and finally, on day four, some skim milk. Because you are consuming too few calories, and far too few calories from carbohydrates, your body believes it is starving, and it kicks into a survival mode (as described above) and weight comes off in a rush.

What have you accomplished? Nothing! You may notice your clothes fitting more loosely, but that's because of lost muscle and water, not fat. And since you lost muscle, you sag more, because the fat is still there. If you have the nerve to stand naked in front of a full length mirror, you'll see exactly what I mean.

And what happens when you start eating like a human being again? The weight comes back! And since your metabolism is depressed (because you lost mostly muscle), you will gain fat at an amazingly rapid rate. Sounds unfair, doesn't it?

Why would any intelligent person go on the cabbage soup diet? The answer is, when it comes to weight loss, the American public is remarkably naive and gullible. We want fast results, and we don't care how we get them. So we try the grapefruit diet, the egg diet, the cucumber diet, the cottage cheese diet, the cabbage soup diet, etc. We lose a bunch of weight, then gain it right back, then move on to the next diet, because it promises to solve our weight problem overnight.

2. WEIGHT LOSS — HOW FAST IS TOO FAST?

I have created a simple test for dieters to predict whether they are losing body fat, or losing muscle. This also predicts whether you will keep off the weight you lost, or gain it right back. This test assumes you are not performing mega-doses of exercise along with your diet, but that you are making an effort to be physically active on a daily basis. The more exercise you do, the more successful you will be in losing body fat and keeping it off. Unfortunately, most dieters don't exercise.

Here is a simple formula (and the table that follows) to rate your efforts in any weight loss program you choose to follow. Use results from the initial phase of your weight loss efforts as a reference point. If your score is high, keep going — you're headed for success. If your score is low, and especially if your score is negative, quit what you're doing and chart a new course.

Ironically, the less weight you lose in the initial phase, the better you are doing, and vice versa. Losing lots of weight quickly virtually guarantees long term failure.

You will use a 30 day reference point which starts after your first week on the diet. You don't use the first week's results, because during this time the body is trying to figure out what's going on. Also, during this very initial phase, even if you are doing everything right, you likely will burn off some stored sugar (glycogen) and lose the water weight that is stored with the sugar. This amounts to anywhere from a 4 to 6 pound weight loss. Obviously, such weight loss is meaningless and misleading. So, your 30 day reference period runs from day 8 to day 38 of your diet.

This approach uses 4 pounds of weight loss per 30 day period as a goal and reference standard. (If you are totally inactive, reduce your goal to only 2 pounds of weight lost in 30 days. All other aspects of the approach, including scoring, stay the same.) Give yourself complete credit for anything up to 4 pounds of weight lost. A 4 pound loss in 30 days earns a score of 4, in other words, and 3 pounds lost in 30 days earns a score of 3, etc.

If you lose more than 4 pounds in the 30 days, you may still be doing okay. Compute the number of pounds over and above the 4 pound standard. The number of pounds above 4 is the "excess." Subtract the excess from 4 to get your score. Here's an example.

If you lost 6 pounds in the 30 day reference period, that's

2 pounds in excess of the standard of 4. Subtract the excess of 2 pounds from 4 and your score is +2. A positive number is a good sign and it means you are doing pretty well. A loss of 7 pounds earns a score of +1. Anything in excess of 7 pounds works against you, as a loss of 8 pounds earns a score of zero, and a loss of more than 8 pounds earns a negative score. Example: 9 pounds minus 4 pounds = 5. 5 is the "excess." Subtract 5 from 4 and the answer is -1.

As you can see, you can earn a score of +2 by losing either 6 pounds or just 2 pounds. Obviously, losing only 2 pounds would entail a more comfortable and easier approach. This is preferable, because the more comfortable you are, the more likely you are to sustain your efforts. Also, losing only 2 pounds of body fat is much better than losing 6 pounds, of which some is fat and some is muscle. As I have written many times, when it comes to losing body fat, zeal is not an asset.

Weight loss	Score	Outcome days 8 - 38
1 to 4 lbs.	+1 to +4	Excellent — Lost weight shouldn't return
5 to 7 lbs	+3 to +1	Good — Lost weight not likely to return
8 to 10 lbs	0 to -2	Not so Good — Lost weight likely to return
11 to 15 lbs	-3 to -7	Bad — Lost weight likely to return quickly
16 lbs and up	-8 and up	Horrible — Lost weight will return like a rocket

The bottom line

The next time someone tells you they are on a new diet and they have lost 12 pounds in just three weeks, smile and say, "I'm sorry to hear that." Maybe this will inspire a conversation that will get them on the right track.

Thermodynamics and crash diets

Any time you shock the body by reducing caloric intake too radically, weight is lost, and the weight that is lost is muscle mass. This is always the explanation for weight that is lost faster than about 1 pound per week. Here's why: According to the first law of thermodynamics, energy is neither created nor destroyed. It can only be transformed. This means, when you are losing weight, you must account for the energy that is transformed. Let's assume you lose 5 pounds in one week (a common occurrence early on when following a bogus diet). You, of course, would like to believe the weight that is lost is body fat. If so, each pound of fat represents 3500 calories (kcals). Can you account for a transformation of 5 times 3500 = 17,500 calories?

The answer is no. A marathon runner can run an entire marathon race (26 miles) and burn off less than 1 pound of fat (about 3250 calories). To date, I haven't come across one single person who is on a high-fat diet who is running the equivalent of about five marathons per week. How, then, is the weight being lost? Easy. The weight is muscle mass which can supply only about 700 usable calories per pound. Thus, it's easy to account for five pounds of muscle loss according to the laws of thermodynamics, because we only have to account for 5 times 700 = 3500 calories for the week.

3. WINNING THE BATTLE OF THE BULGE

Everywhere you turn these days, it seems that the news surrounding our battle with the bulge is bleak. We're too fat, getting fatter year by year, and getting fatter faster. Yikes! Seems like eventually we'll all be homebound, because we'll be so fat we won't be able to get out the door. Not really.

Fortunately, some are doing well and actually are winning the battle of the bulge. They are a lot fewer in number, of course, than those who are losing the battle. But the mere fact that there are some winners out there is encouraging, and suggests that if you put your mind to it, you can win too.

The National Weight Control Registry is an ongoing research study which keeps track of those who successfully lose weight and keep it off. To qualify, you must have lost at least 30 pounds and have kept it off for at least one year. It's possible that you might have lost more than 30 pounds and gained some back, but you are eligible if your net loss is at least 30 pounds. To date, the average person in the registry has lost about 60 pounds and has kept it off five years.

Much has been learned

Much has been learned about the thousands of successful individuals in the registry which can help us understand the causes of obesity, and possibly create solutions. For example, more than 75 percent were obese young in life, prior to the age of 18, and the majority were obese already by the age of 11.

Over 70 percent have at least one parent who is obese, suggesting a genetic link. This is an interesting finding, because those with a genetic link tend to throw their hands in the air and admit failure, believing they are powerless to overcome their heredity. The fact that so many in the registry are successful in shedding pounds and keeping them off demonstrates that gumption and know-how can overcome genetics.

A key finding is that most were yo-yo dieters at one time or another, losing weight, then gaining it back, and losing it again. This means, even though you may have a past history of failure, keep trying and eventually you will succeed.

What weight reduction program is best? About half of registrants were helped by organized programs such as Weight Watchers and Overeaters Anonymous, and by psychological counseling (one on one, or group), while the other half were successful on their own. The difference between men and women is interesting. Typically, men were inspired to change for health reasons, while the trigger for women was emotional and wanting to feel better about themselves.

Rules of thumb for success

There were a number of common "rules of thumb" among successful registrants.

1. Nine out of ten changed *both* their eating and their

exercise habits. This underscores what I have been saying for years. What you put in your mouth is the decisive factor in the battle, but you won't be truly successful in managing your weight unless you are more physically active on a daily basis. Registrants report doing lots of moderate exercise, most expending as much as 400 calories per day (equivalent to walking about 4 miles, or performing other moderate physical activities for approximately one hour).

2. Very few of the registrants used fad diets. They couldn't, and still be successful in the long run. You now know why.

3. Typical successful strategies include eating frequent and smaller meals, avoiding fast food restaurants, cutting back on fat intake, and cutting portion sizes — all common sense approaches.

4. Registrants report that keeping the weight off is easier than losing it in the first place. That's because they have taken a sane and long term approach to their weight loss. Those on a crash diet report the opposite — taking the weight off is easy compared to keeping it off. On a crash diet, they victimize themselves with an extreme approach which causes them to quickly lose many pounds of muscle and water. That's the easy part. But once you do this, it's virtually impossible to sustain this unnatural state, so the weight comes back on in a rush.

5. One factor surprised me. Some successful registrants weigh themselves frequently, at least once a week, and some weigh every day. I am against this, because it puts too much pressure on you and doesn't allow for natural ups and downs. Regardless, some find it helpful.

6. Finally, it's nice to know that these successful individuals feel good about their transition and that they are not miserable, nor do they feel as if they are engaged in a constant struggle. They have changed their lifestyle to the point where their lifestyle is working for them, making it easy to sustain their weight loss. What's more, they report feeling so much better than they used to, which is a strong stimulus to continue.

4. PLATEAUS DURING WEIGHT LOSS

Usually, plateaus are not really plateaus, but rather are periods when weight loss slows down so much that it appears as if nothing is happening. When this occurs and when you compare a reduced rate of weight loss with a former faster rate, you become discouraged. If you ride it out and take a long-range view (as every investment broker advises for your stock market portfolio) you will see continued progress.

Plateaus are particularly discouraging to those on a crash diet. When you are doing things wrong and losing weight too fast, you plateau quickly because your body cannot sustain such a rapid rate of loss. On a crash diet you will lose several pounds (as many as five or six) in the first few days. This is because you are losing stored carbohydrate (glycogen) and the water that is stored with it. Once this is gone, you experience your first plateau (a substantial reduction in the rate of weight loss).

If you keep going, you begin breaking down your muscles and converting the proteins to fuel. Again, this will proceed rapidly (a pound of weight loss every few days) for a while, then slow down again. Eventually, because you are literally starving yourself and losing muscle mass, your metabolism will plummet which will prevent you from losing so much muscle so quickly. You enter another plateau, in other words.

This is the point at which most people abandon their insane crash diet. The contrast of losing so much so fast leads to unrealistic expectations. Then, when things slow down, disappointment sets in and you stop. Thank goodness. The loss of stored carbohydrate, water, and muscle does you no good at all, and can endanger your health. Stopping is the best thing you can do. Unfortunately, the moment you stop, the weight comes back on in a hurry. But you tend to gain back fat, even though you didn't lose much fat on the diet. It's not fair, is it? No, but that's the way it is.

Legitimate plateaus

If you are doing things right, you can avoid the plateaus described above, but ultimately you will probably encounter plateaus somewhere along the line. Because you are doing the right things, let's call these legitimate plateaus. Here's what may be happening to slow even a good weight loss program.

Let's assume for argument's sake that you start a weight loss program weighing 285 pounds, and you reduce your caloric intake to a level commensurate with sustaining the bodyweight of someone weighing 200 pounds. Originally, before dieting, you were consuming enough calories to sustain 285 pounds, so this would be a substantial reduction. Over a prolonged period of time, you will lose weight. But as you go along, the rate will get slower and slower, especially as you approach 200 pounds. There are two reason for this. As you change in size, getting smaller, your metabolism will decrease. In addition, as you approach a bodyweight of 200 pounds, your diet gradually shifts away from weight loss and toward maintenance, because your caloric intake is designed to support 200 pounds. (More on this in Chapter 6.)

If metabolism is declining, is it smart to reduce caloric intake further? Maybe. But, sometimes this can be a problem, because reducing caloric intake too much can reduce metabolism even further. This means, ironically, you could find yourself in a position of not consuming enough calories to continue losing body fat. This sounds strange, I know, but it's a fact.

So, what should you do when a plateau occurs? Relax, be patient, don't panic, and don't do anything radical and silly. Ride it out for a few months and you probably will see the loss of a few additional pounds. If not, visit a dietitian to examine your diet and make healthful recommendations. Increase your daily exercise to give your metabolism a boost. A great addition is resistance training to build muscle mass. It's possible in the early stages of a diet, especially a crash diet, that you may lose a considerable amount of muscle mass. Gaining back some muscle will increase your metabolism, even at rest.

The bottom line is that losing body fat is a long-range

process. Plateaus may be part of the process, but that's pretty typical of life in general, isn't it? Things rarely flow smoothly from beginning to end. Anticipate the rough spots, keep doing the right things, and eventually you will be successful.

5. HOW MUCH SHOULD YOU WEIGH?

I can take you into my laboratory and with sophisticated methodologies determine your body fat percentage. From there I can determine a weight that will give you a desirable percentage of body fat. This would be your target weight. But since you don't have access to these resources, we'll go to plan B. Simply determine the weight you want to be. When you do, and assuming you use good common sense, you'll probably be very close to your target weight — a weight that's right for you.

A good reference point is your weight when you were a young adult (approximately 21 years of age) plus approximately 3 percent for each decade beyond your twenties, up to a total of 10 percent. If you are in your thirties, you would add 3 percent to the weight you were as a young adult, add 6 percent if you are in your forties, and no more than 10 percent in your fifties and beyond. This assumes, of course, that you were satisfied with your weight as a young adult. If you weighed 150 pounds at age 21, your limits would be approximately 155 in your 30's, 160 in your 40's, and 165 in your 50's and beyond.

If you were not satisfied with your weight as a young adult, obviously you don't want to use that weight as a target. Instead, subtract a reasonable number of pounds from your present weight. If your weight has been a problem for many years, you probably have a good idea of how many pounds need to come off.

How many calories and fat grams should you consume?
In order to reach your target weight, the best approach is to eat the number of calories and fat grams that will sustain that weight. If you are satisfied with your present weight, your present

weight is your target. But, since you are likely to be heavier than your target weight, eating in accordance with the level of energy required to sustain your target weight (and not your present weight) will cause you to lose weight gradually.

For example, if you currently weigh 200 pounds and your target is 160 pounds, you eventually will weigh 160 pounds if you consume only the amount of energy required to sustain that weight. Obviously, the amount of energy required to sustain 160 pounds is less than that required to sustain 200 pounds, and the difference between the two will represent the degree to which you drop your caloric intake from its present level. The process will be very slow, but that's okay. Remember, in the ultimate, it's the tortoise who wins the race, not the hare.

To determine how many calories and fat grams to consume, consult the tables below. Calories are listed according to your target weight, and take into account four different levels of physical activity. The number of fat grams you will consume are included in parentheses. The fat content represents approximately 15-17 percent of total calories. Note: Keep your grams of saturated fat to as near zero as possible.

If you are over 30 years of age, round your target weight down to a weight included in the table. This means if you are 31 years old or older and your target weight is 127, you would round down to 120. Rounding down will help compensate for the gradual reduction in metabolic rate that occurs with aging. If you are 30 years of age or below, round to the nearest weight (127 would round to 130, for example, and 124 rounds to 120).

Choose your typical level of daily physical activity from one of the four categories below. If in doubt about which category is yours, err on the conservative side and take the lower activity level. Most people will be in the first two categories. Enter the column in the table under the physical activity label you select and find your target weight. This is the number of calories (and fat grams in parentheses) you should consume.

There is more on the Jack Sprat plan ahead. This approach is the basis for my Jack Sprat Low-fat Diet Plan.

DEFINITIONS:

Couch potato: You specialize in avoiding physical activity and limit yourself to things like walking short distances to and from your car — to the office or the house — and once inside, your movement is limited. Evenings and weekends are more likely to find you in front of the TV than outside.

Mild activity: You don't go out of your way to add exercise to your life, but you don't avoid it either. You are somewhat active on the job and/or around the house. This means you spend at least a portion of the work day on your feet — frequently running errands on the job (several times per hour). At home, you engage in typical household chores. Weekends find you outside at least part of the time, in the garden, walking in the park, washing the car, cutting the grass, engaging in light sporting activities such as golf, doubles tennis, etc.

Moderate activity: In addition to the items associated with "mild activity," you incorporate exercise into your daily routine for approximately one hour per day. The exercise is brisk, but not terribly demanding — brisk walking or light jogging, aerobics classes, moderate sporting activities such as basketball, squash or singles tennis. On weekends you are likely to be very physically active. A highly active job, such as being a waitress, carpenter, delivery person, etc. in which you are on your feet and moving continually will get you into this category.

Heavy activity: If you engage in heavy aerobic training (running an hour or more per day) or if you are employed in heavy industry (construction, foundry work, etc.), you will require a substantial number of calories to sustain your weight. But this category should be reserved only for those who perform intensive and prolonged exercise on a daily basis.

TABLE 1 WOMEN

DAILY CALORIC INTAKE (FAT GRAMS)

Target Weight	Couch Potato	Mild Activity	Moderate Activity	Heavy Activity
100	1410 (23)	1570 (26)	1880 (31)	2190 (37)
110	1460 (24)	1620 (27)	1940 (32)	2270 (38)
120	1510 (25)	1670 (28)	2010 (33)	2340 (39)
130	1560 (26)	1730 (29)	2070 (34)	2420 (40)
140	1610 (27)	1790 (30)	2150 (36)	2510 (42)
150	1650 (28)	1840 (31)	2200 (37)	2570 (43)
160	1710 (29)	1900 (32)	2280 (38)	2660 (44)
170	1760 (30)	1960 (33)	2350 (39)	2740 (46)
180	1800 (31)	2000 (34)	2400 (40)	2800 (47)
190	1850 (32)	2050 (35)	2460 (41)	2870 (48)
200	1890 (33)	2090 (36)	2510 (42)	2930 (49)

TABLE 2 MEN

DAILY CALORIC INTAKE (FAT GRAMS)

Target Weight	Couch Potato	Mild Activity	Moderate Activity	Heavy Activity
120	1640 (27)	1820 (30)	2180 (36)	2550 (43)
130	1700 (28)	1890 (31)	2260 (38)	2640 (44)
140	1760 (29)	1950 (32)	2340 (39)	2740 (46)
150	1820 (30)	2020 (33)	2420 (40)	2830 (47)
160	1860 (31)	2070 (34)	2480 (41)	2890 (48)
170	1910 (32)	2120 (35)	2540 (42)	2970 (49)
180	1960 (33)	2180 (36)	2610 (43)	3040 (51)
190	2000 (34)	2220 (37)	2660 (44)	3110 (52)
200	2040 (35)	2260 (38)	2720 (45)	3170 (53)
210	2100 (36)	2330 (39)	2800 (46)	3260 (54)
220	2140 (37)	2380 (40)	2850 (47)	3320 (55)
230	2180 (38)	2420 (41)	2900 (48)	3390 (56)
240	2210 (39)	2450 (42)	2940 (49)	3430 (57)

The Jack Sprat Low Fat Diet

I created the Jack-Sprat Low-fat Diet with my co-author, Becca Coffin, RN. (*The Jack Sprat Low-fat Diet: A 28-day Heart Healthy Plan You Can Follow the Rest of Your Life* — University Press of Kentucky, 1995.) Our purpose in creating it was to address the insanity which envelopes the weight management world, and to have a useful tool when working with our weight- loss clients. I hated to use the word "diet" in the title, because Jack Sprat is so much more than a diet book. Moreover, it's not a diet, at least not the kind of diet most Americans are accustomed to experiencing. It is a healthy eating plan which can lead to sustained reductions in body fatness.

The Jack Sprat approach is different in many ways. First, the plan is grounded in reality. A guiding principle when we put the Jack Sprat plan together was, what are people willing to do everyday and for the rest of their lives? If something struck us as trendy or transient, we didn't include it. If you don't make changes that are comfortable and that you intend to keep, what's the point? Temporary weight loss does no one any good.

Unlike the hundreds of diet plans available in book stores, we won't promise quick weight loss. On the contrary, we promise a slow and steady loss (about one pound per week). Doesn't sound very exciting, does it? It isn't, but it's the only way to be successful in the long run.

As I have stated repeatedly, to emphasize its extreme importance, crash diets quickly cause weight loss because you are losing muscle and water. On Jack Sprat, you lose more slowly, because you are losing body fat. If it were possible to lose fat in a hurry, you would be capable of quickly stripping away your vital energy reserves, a fact that would have led to our demise as a species long ago when food was less plentiful and famine was a constant threat.

The Jack Sprat plan is both a weight reduction and weight maintenance program. This is important because most people who diet and reach their target weight regain the weight within the first year. One reason is, they don't know how to shift from a weight reduction diet to a maintenance diet. On Jack Sprat, no shift is necessary, and there is no need to change the way you eat when you reach your target weight.

The amount of food you eat will surprise you. It's a lot, and it's not just to help you be comfortable and feel good about what you are doing. Ironically, if you don't consume enough food, you cannot lose fat from your body. Most women who see the Jack Sprat plan for the first time are amazed at the amount of food they are told to eat. They say they've never eaten that much. The reason you can eat so much is the low fat content of the plan — only 15-17 percent of the calories come from fat, and almost none of the fat is saturated fat.

The carbohydrates in Jack Sprat are the healthy complex type which don't cause the insulin problems associated with simple sugars. Jack Sprat is not just another low-fat, high-sugar diet, in other words. That's not to say there are not treats involved in the diet. There are, but they are used sparingly.

There are detailed menus in which we tell you exactly what to eat, meal by meal, for 28 days. Easy to fix and tasty low-fat recipes are provided. Grocery lists are included for each of the four weeks. Take the list to your supermarket and buy everything on the list and you will have what you need for the week. We have plenty of exchanges built in which allow you to drop food items you don't like and add others while staying within the Jack Sprat guidelines.

We realize no one can stick to a diet everyday, no matter how comfortable it is. You are going to want to cheat, and we'll help you. We have incorporated "Warthog" days in which you can eat the things that got you in trouble in the first place. Things like giant hamburgers, pizza, fried chicken, tacos and the like are included within a context that doesn't penalize you too severely. You can't cheat everyday, obviously, but it's nice to know that when you need to cheat you can. And after you cheat, you can get right back on the plan without missing a beat.

In a nutshell, the Jack Sprat plan offers a generous dose of common sense mixed with tried and proven scientific principles. It's not glitzy or glamorous, and it won't transform you overnight from a frog to a prince. But it works. You can purchase (or order) copies of the Jack Sprat Low-fat diet at bookstores, or order directly from the University Press of Kentucky (1-800-839-6855). In addition, if you would like assistance in your weight loss efforts (regardless of what plan you are following), feel free to call the Health Promotion Center at 502-852-5711 I will be glad to help you in any way I can.

6. EATING RIGHT IS NOT AS HARD AS YOU THINK

The purpose of this book is to point you in the right direction, and to provide you with a sane philosophy you can depend on to take you where you want to go. As I've said, it is not intended to be a precise and detailed diet book. I've done that already when I wrote The Jack Sprat Low-fat Diet. But if you want to make some useful and sustainable changes, there is much you can do on your own right now. In fact, chances are good you already know of lots of things you could, and should, be doing. Let's review some of them.

Change your attitude
Somewhere along the line, the majority of Americans have adopted the mistaken notion that it is their birthright to eat whatever they want and in whatever amounts they choose. Indeed, they feel truly put upon when told that regularly consuming bacon cheeseburgers, fries, prime rib, donuts, etc. is a dangerous thing to do. Some listen, however, and believe what they hear, but still they won't give up these foods because they taste too good. It's obvious that doing what is preferred rather than what is prudent and needed dominates the choice of what we eat in this country.

This approach is less likely in other areas of life. There is a pile of bills on your desk that need to be paid, and you know late fees are right around the corner if you don't act now. You pay the bills rather than take a nap. Obviously, you are aware that it is not your birthright to ignore these things and do what is pleasurable instead. The reason is, there are consequences to pay that are immediately apparent to you.

That's not to say there are no consequences from eating poorly. On the contrary, eating poorly sets the stage for the most devastating of consequences. But we don't see them, because the consequences are delayed and typically don't show themselves for decades. Thus, over the years we fool ourselves into believing we are getting away with it. We're not, and the epidemic of obesity and the widespread chronic diseases which disable and kill us scream this message loud and clear.

In order to make any meaningful and long lasting change, you must first adopt a positive attitude about change. Yes, it will take effort and sacrifice. Anything worthwhile has these costs. But once you are over the hump and have moved the changes into the mainstream of your lifestyle, you'll look back in disbelief about the health destroying things you used to do.

Recognize and avoid dietary villains

If you were to cut way back on the big three dietary villains, your weight management efforts would take a quantum leap forward, and your health profile would benefit greatly.

Saturated fat — Dietary fat makes you fat, and saturated fat is the worst form of fat. Saturated fat is public enemy number one, contributing to many devastating effects in your body, including boosting your serum cholesterol. Your body does not require saturated fat, so it's best to set a goal of zero intake. Such a goal may not be possible for everyone, but if you can come anywhere close to this, your body will thank you.

Anything you can do to reduce the intake of this killer will pay huge health dividends for you. Fortunately, it's easy to recognize saturated fat and easy to confront. But to overcome it won't be easy, because you'll have to make the conscious decision to overrule your taste buds. Unfortunately, things that taste good often taste good because they are loaded with saturated fat.

Food labels tell you how much saturated fat is contained in foods per serving. Focus your attention on avoiding the leading sources of saturated fat: 1. ground beef (hamburgers, meatloaf); 2. processed meats (wieners, bologna, salami); 3. fatty dairy products (cheese, whole milk, ice cream); 4. baked goods (donuts, croissants, cakes, pies); and, 5. cuts of meat (roasts, steaks, ribs). Add to this list the process of frying in oils loaded with saturated fat (beef tallow and south of the border oils such as coconut, palm and palm kernel oils) and you get a massive dose of saturated fat daily if you eat like a typical American.

Sugar — Sugar, because of its effects to evoke a huge insulin response, has seized center stage along with dietary fat as co-conspirators to help make you fat. The reason is, insulin helps you store fat. What's more, excess sugar calories are converted to body fat. Both these factors make avoiding sugar as important as avoiding dietary fat.

Sugar is a broad term that covers good and bad sugars. Good sugars are complex in nature (meaning they break down slowly during digestion, which reduces the body's insulin response). Good sugars are complex carbs which include the prime components of most diets in the world—rice, whole grain products, vegetables, beans and corn, potatoes, and pasta.

Simple sugars are bad (because they break down quickly during digestion and cause a huge insulin response). Simple sugars are found in abundance in products that contain table sugar, including candy and sweets of any kind, cakes, pies, cookies, etc. White processed (enriched) flour is another culprit. For most Americans the best way to reduce simple sugar intake dramatically is to avoid softdrinks which contain many teaspoons of sugar per 12-ounce can.

Sugar is devastating to those with insulin resistance. Insulin resistance is found most often in the obese and it means the cells of the body resist the effects of insulin to move sugar into the cells. The result is the build-up of sugar in the blood stream and an attempt by the body to fix this problem by overproducing insulin. Both excess sugar and excess insulin are devastating to the body over time. Unfortunately, millions of Americans are walking around with excess sugar and insulin in their blood and they don't know it. What's worse, their daily diet exaggerates the problem because of the high sugar intake.

Salt — Although salt is not a major player when it comes to weight management, it has great importance when it comes to overall health. A high salt intake can contribute to high blood pressure — "the silent killer." Some people (about 20 percent of the population) are highly salt sensitive, but research suggests that all of us would benefit from a substantial reduction in salt intake. Sodium is the culprit in salt, so keep your eye on the sodium content on food labels and shoot for a total of less than 2000 mg of sodium per day — the lower the better. Most of us take in much more than this.

Eat fresh foods

Most of us have gotten so used to eating processed foods (canned, boxed, dried, frozen, pre-prepared) that we forget about fresh fruits, vegetables and whole grain products. Too bad, because processed foods are loaded with fat and the two most popular additives, sugar and salt. Shifting your attention to fresh foods is a great way to avoid these killers.

Fresh foods offer additional benefits. They are an excellent source of nutrients that may be absent in processed foods, and fresh vegetables rank number one in potential nutrient value. Processing can kill valuable vitamins, and it's only recently that we discovered the value of phytochemicals (nutrients in plants that have functions similar to vitamins) and antioxidants that are found in abundance in fresh vegetables. Fresh vegetables also are a valuable source of fiber.

Learn to appreciate the flavors of fresh foods without adding butter and salt. It may take a while to retrain your taste buds, but it can be done and it's not as difficult as it may seem at first. All it takes is commitment. Learning to drink skim milk rather than whole milk, for example, takes commitment. At first, skim milk tastes like dish water. But eventually, you adjust, and once you have made the shift, you never want to go back to whole milk again, because it's thickness and high fat content will turn you off.

Eat less

To lose weight, eat less. This is obvious, and it's true regardless of what you eat. But there's more to the story.

Considerable research on animals shows that eating less contributes to a longer and healthier life. Most experts believe this is true for humans as well. Eating less is challenging, because in order to do so safely, you must choose your foods more carefully, getting more nutrient value per calorie ingested. This leaves no room for empty calories such as soft drinks and snack foods which provide hundreds of calories with absolutely no nutrient value whatsoever.

Here are a few tips. To eat less, eat more slowly. When you have finished a meal and are still hungry, take a break and allow some time before eating more. Divert your attention and often you will find that the hunger disappears and that you feel fully satisfied. Pay attention to when and where you eat. Eat only at the dinner table, and quit grabbing food from the refrigerator or the cupboard. Eat lower calorie foods which allow more volume and satisfy you more quickly.

My strategy for eating less

Those who have been reading my column over the years know that in the old days my diet was deplorable. It changed about 14 years ago for the better, and today, I am a qualified vegetarian. That means I am not a vegan (one who eats nothing of animal origin), but rather, I eat fish and consume egg whites.

Until recently, I have regularly consumed very large quantities of food. But, knowing that eating less is a healthy thing to do, I have cut back on my food intake. Also, as I get older, I don't burn calories as fast as I used to, and if I'm not careful I'll add weight easily. As I cut back my volume, I have found that I feel so much better throughout the day. This makes sense. When you bring food into the body, you place a stress on the body to digest it, absorb it and assimilate the components into the cells. This takes precious energy, and it imposes a wear and tear factor on all the physiologic machinery involved in the process.

As a strategy, I eat very little in the morning, but I make certain I eat something. I find that if I eat a lot of carbs in the morning I feel less energetic as the morning progresses, and I'm much hungrier by lunch time. This feeling was not always the case, but as I get older, the effect is increasingly noticeable. To combat this, for breakfast I eat some soy cheese and a handful of raw nuts, usually walnuts. (Be careful here, because nuts are high in calories and fat, but the fat is good monounsaturated fat.) I know what you're thinking — Ugh! — but the combination is really quite tasty and satisfying. And, it takes no preparation time and can be consumed while you are doing all the other things you do on busy mornings.

Because of my light intake of food in the morning and the low intake of carbohydrates (causing a low insulin response), I feel satisfied and energetic and the feeling stays for quite some time. This type of morning eating with a low carb (sugar) intake would be particularly helpful for those who are insulin-resistant. (Note: Most who are overweight, especially those with considerable abdominal fat stores, are at least a little insulin-resistant).

I don't even think about eating again until late in the morning when hunger visits. When it does I'll usually turn to carbs, and have some fruit (a grapefruit, pear, banana), and a high nutrient (protein/carb) bar.

Later, I may or may not have lunch. I leave it to how I feel. A key here is that I'm not locked into eating, but rather I allow my body to tell me what to do. If I have lunch, I prepare it and eat it in my office. I'll microwave a couple of soy chicken patties, soy hot dogs, or soy burgers and put them on whole grain bread with mustard and relish. Very tasty! I avoid eating out, because that's where you can really get into trouble, especially on a daily basis. A good rule of thumb is, where possible, choose brown bagging it over eating out, because bringing your own lunch gives you control over what you eat and in what portions. I may have a healthful snack in mid- to late afternoon.

Dinner is my main meal and I don't hold back, especially now that I have Anita, my fiance, a dietitian who loves to cook, prepping my vittles. Eating a pretty hefty amount of food once a day at dinner satisfies my desire to load up, but because it's only once a day, rather than twice or three times, the overall effect on the quantity I eat per day is not great.

Once or twice a week we'll have fish. Otherwise, we eat lots of soy products (buffalo wings, chicken nuggets, garden burgers, etc.), healthy homemade pizza with lots of tomato sauce and vegetables, burritos with lots of vegetables, different types of whole grain pastas, vegetarian lasagna, vegetable soups and chili, etc. Depending on what we eat, I'll pack away a fair amount of whole grain bread with my meal. Sometimes there may be low-fat cheese included in some things I eat. While I tend to avoid this, I'm not so fanatical in my approach that I feel like a traitor to my vegetarian leanings.

There also are many times when as a meal I'll make a blend of soy milk, soy protein powder, egg-beaters, and fruit. Or, I may have nothing more than a large bowl of whole grain cereal or oatmeal with fruit and soy milk, or a sandwich with natural peanut butter on whole grain bread.

As you can see, my diet is pretty simple most of the time, and my day is structured so that I'm not tempted to overindulge myself and eat a lot of food. Although I tend to eat a fairly large amount for dinner, when considering my overall food intake for the day, it's not all that much. Thinking back to my old ways of eating, the saying "I wish I'd known then what I know now," comes to mind. But it's never too late to start feeling good and to be healthier.

Eat mindfully
Some day I'll tackle my next goal of eating mindfully.

That is, paying close attention to what you are eating. Most of us don't. Our eating is automatic, and we tend to gulp things down as if there were no tomorrow. Admittedly, I'm guilty of eating this way, and I know if I were to slow down and pay more attention, I'd enjoy my food more. I'd also probably eat even less, a continuing goal of mine. At least I am aware of what I need to be doing. That's an important first step. And, occasionally I do eat mindfully, and when I do I feel good about it. That's an important second step. Eventually, I'll take more steps and incorporate this into my lifestyle.

Daily inventory

In a friendly and gentle way, check in on yourself with a personal inventory. People in business, and those in sales, in particular, are taught to do this. At the end of the day, they recount how they did. Did they accomplish everything they intended? If not, they vow to do better. If they did, they experience reinforcement and a sense of satisfaction. This is an excellent way to stay on track. I suggest modifying this notion by taking a daily health and weight management inventory. At the end of the day, ask yourself: Did I contribute to my health and weight management today, or did I do the opposite. Specifically, did I eat right, or eat wrong?

If it was a bad day, acknowledge it and let it go. If it was a good day, bask in the achievement and success and use it to reinforce your efforts. Keep in mind that the ultimate results you achieve will be the sum total of your daily efforts.

The bottom line

With the possible exception of quitting cigarette smoking, eating right is the most important thing you can do for your health and to assist you in your weight management efforts. To get started in the right direction, change your attitude and accept that change may require some effort and sacrifice. Next, focus your attention on one of my suggestions and stick with it until you have conquered it. Then move on. Eventually, your diet will be working for you, instead of working against you.

7. HIGH-FAT DIETS AND LOW-SUGAR DIETS

Inevitably, when I log onto my computer each day, I can count on at least one e-mail question, and often several, regarding the benefits of a high-fat diet. There is an insatiable hunger for a magic bullet when it comes to weight loss, and the high-fat diet is the latest in a long line of pretenders.

As I have said many times, there are lots of things you can do to lose weight in a hurry, including going on a high fat binge. Here's how it works. When you load up on fat, and keep the carbohydrates low, the body can't process all the fat that's coming in. The fats are broken down to their component parts resulting in the release of fatty acids. When there are too many fatty acids being formed, they accumulate, creating acidosis, a dangerous condition which can cause you to lapse into a coma. Fortunately, the liver provides an outlet, preventing acidosis, at least for a while. It takes the fatty acids and creates ketone bodies (also called ketones).

This is only a temporary solution, however. The accumulation of ketones (a condition called ketosis) also is dangerous, because ketones are acidic and can contribute to acidosis. When ketones build up excessively, they spill over into the urine (a condition known as ketonuria). Important minerals (sodium and potassium) are excreted along with the ketones, creating a mineral imbalance and contributing to acidosis. Symptoms including dizziness, fatigue, nausea and vomiting may accompany ketosis.

You *can* consume large amounts of fatty food and still lose weight. These circumstances are similar to that of people who cannot use carbohydrates as fuel, because there is not sufficient insulin to escort glucose into the cells. In other words, the high fat diet forces your body to operate in the same kind of desperate circumstances as those with uncontrolled diabetes.

As if that isn't bad enough, too much fat intake can lead to high levels of uric acid in the blood. This can be a serious problem because uric acid levels may already be high in heavy individuals, and a high-fat diet could compound this, possibly leading to an attack of gouty arthritis. In addition, a high fat intake generally means a high intake of saturated fat. Saturated fat is damaging to the body in many ways, including the promotion of LDL-cholesterol production in the liver.

There are other aspects of this insane diet which guarantee it's failure. Fat takes a long time to digest, and this makes you less hungry. Ketone bodies also suppress appetite. Thus, eventually, you may begin eating less, even though you are already starving yourself. As you starve, you break down proteins from your muscles, losing muscle while your body fat remains intact. The fact that you are losing weight fast is exciting, of course. But it wouldn't be if you knew what was happening inside your body and that you were losing large amounts of muscle mass.

High fat diets emphasize meat and dairy intake, and therefore they are also high in protein. Excessive protein intake leads to nitrogen waste products which must be handled by your kidneys. Too much of this can overwork the kidneys. Healthy kidneys can probably handle the load, but those with unknown kidney problems can be thrown over the edge. Too much dietary protein can cause uremic poisoning (the accumulation of toxic waste products due to kidney failure). Excess protein, especially from animal sources (meat and dairy products), also pulls calcium from your bones, contributing to osteoporosis.

The fact that in some cases physicians have recommended this unhealthy diet to patients prior to surgery is not an endorsement. Rather, in some cases, it is necessary to get weight off quickly by whatever means possible. I once endorsed a crazy crash diet (not the high-fat diet) for a friend who was suffering terribly from lower back pain. I knew that reducing her size would help, regardless of whether she lost muscle or body fat. She took off nearly 90 pounds and her back felt better. Unfortunately, she didn't learn any sustainable healthy eating habits during the diet.

And, because she lost the weight quickly and most of what she lost was muscle and water, she quickly gained back what she lost (and more) once she returned to her old ways of eating. The back problem returned with a vengeance, too.

A major problem with high-fat diets is that you become accustomed to eating lots of fat early in the diet, when the notion of loading up on fatty treats is appealing. But, eventually, you realize that fatty foods are not nearly as palatable when carbs are missing. Eating eggs without toast, for example, or prime rib without a baked potato. When the newness wears off, it's very likely you will begin incorporating carbs back into your diet. It's natural — your body will be screaming for them. But you won't cut your fat, because you mistakenly believe that all that fat intake is okay. And since you used to eat carbs loaded with simple sugar, those are the kind you bring back into your diet. Eventually, then, you are not only back where you started from, but now you are consuming way too much fat. Is it any wonder that the backlash weight gain is tremendous?

A reader writes
I went on a high fat diet for about three weeks. At first, it was great, the most wonderful diet in the world. I ate red meat, bacon, cheese, sour cream, butter, fried everything, and the pounds melted off. I was in heaven. What's more, I lost my appetite. At first, I thought this was great, too. But then I realized that the thought of eating made me a little nauseated. I didn't want to chew on another piece of meat or a hunk of cheese. The thought of another "delicacy" of tuna wrapped in American cheese made me gag. But I kept going, and as I did I realized how hollow this fantasy was. Sure, I could eat sour cream, but on what? How was I supposed to enjoy all this butter I could eat — lather it on steak? Realizing how deprived I really was, I began to cheat and, of course, things fell apart quickly. Other people who have been on this crazy diet scheme have experienced the same thing. Eating like that seems wonderful at first, but be careful of what you wish for. You just might get it.

My response

This story is a familiar one. Returning to carbs is always the ruin of a high-fat diet, and everyone will return to carbs sooner or later. Thus, such plans always are doomed. Fortunately, when you go on these crazy diets you can't stay on them for long. The wisdom of the body recognizes the unhealthy aspects of the diet and the body won't let you continue. That's why I don't try to intervene when friends and acquaintances get excited and jump on the high-fat crash diet bandwagon. Instead, I encourage them to come see me in a year or so and show me the long-term benefits of their efforts. To date, not one person has ever come back in one year to discuss the wondrous effects of their magic bullet diet. In fact, it's typical that, should I run into them, they are firmly silent on the issue, embarrassed, knowing the weight they have gained back says it all.

A reader writes

I have been on a high-fat diet for several months. I am not only losing weight, my health is better. My cholesterol is down, my blood pressure is down and I feel better. If, as you say, high fat diets are so bad, why do they seem to help? Lately, I have switched to an insulin control diet, and I am still feeling great. Please comment.

My response

I have received many responses to my high-fat diet column, and several are similar to yours. By that I mean they are well thought out and make a number of good points. Many, on the other hand, are merely testimonies from those who have been on such diets for a short term and have lost a lot of weight and who therefore are misled into believing they are being successful. I tend to disregard such responses, because soon they will realize their efforts are foolhardy, and that following their rapid weight loss there is rapid weight gain.

The vast majority of responses to what I wrote have been favorable. Many have related their own experiences or those of friends who have suffered negative consequences from overloading on fat. As such, I am firm in my belief that high-fat diets should be condemned, and I stand by the many reasons I cited previously.

I realize, of course, that my stance and letters such as yours beg the questions: 1. If low-fat diets are so good, why do bad things happen on these diets? 2. If high-fat diet are so awful, why do so many people seem to realize positive health outcomes? The answers to these questions are quite simple, and, in fact, your letter underscores several additional points which must be made to clarify this situation.

The answer to the first question is this: Low-fat diets often are actually high-sugar diets that are as unhealthy as high-fat diets. Low-fat diets are supposed to be healthy. They help you lose weight and improve your health profile. Pretty clear cut, right? I used to think so. But lately, low-fat diets have come under assault by those who claim that dietary fat is not the problem. It's sugar. Some low-fat bashers have gone so far as to say that dietary fat is healthy and you should eat as much as you like. Indeed, I've been bombarded with comments from those on high-fat diets who gloat that they've lost inches and pounds while wolfing down bacon, cheeseburgers and fries. Are they telling the truth? Yes. How is that possible?

At the core is the fact that not all low-fat diets are good for you. Some, as pointed out by the low-fat bashers, are downright bad. A bad low-fat diet is one that is low in fat, but high in sugar. This is a natural outgrowth of myopic vision which focuses attention entirely on dietary fat as the only culprit in the diet. When this happens, the thrust is to reduce dietary fat at any cost, even if it means loading up on sugary treats to compensate the loss of taste from reducing fat intake.

Thus, the low-fat diet has become the high-sugar diet, and too much sugar causes problems. The body's exaggerated insulin response is the key. Thus, when the high sugar diet is abandoned, even in favor of lots of dietary fat and protein, some good things can happen.

The answer to the second question is: It's the low sugar intake that helps, not the high fat. You cut back on sugar, and in the process you also reduced your caloric intake — both of which are highly positive. Furthermore, I submit, the healthy changes you have observed were made *in spite of* the high fat intake, and *not because of it*!

One final point, and I believe this says it all. According to your letter, you followed the high-fat diet for only several months, then switched to the insulin control diet (a balanced diet that includes lots of complex carbs). Why would you switch if you truly believed the high-fat diet you were on was, in the long run, beneficial to your health? I suspect you quit the high-fat diet for the same reason everyone else does. Your body rebels and lets you know you'd better quit, or else.

To your great credit, instead of quitting and going back to your old habits, you switched to the diet you are now on, the insulin control diet. I applaud your choice. But the point remains, your experiences on the high-fat diet were limited in terms of longevity, and certainly did not represent a meaningful change in lifestyle. Moreover, you wisely gave up that diet, and the fact that you have been able to sustain your weight loss is due to the fact that now you are following a more realistic and healthful diet. Even so, chances are good that you lost considerable muscle mass on the high-fat diet that accounts for a good portion of total weight you lost and this, of course, needs to be replaced.

The bottom line is, a low-fat and high-sugar diet is bad for you. I yield on this point and support criticism of the insulin inducing effects of such a diet. A high-fat and low-sugar diet is bad for you, too. A low-fat and high-complex carbohydrate diet is the best choice, and this is what I advocate. As a compromise, a moderate-fat (no saturated fat) and high-complex carbohydrate diet is not a bad choice, and may be perceived by many Americans as being more user-friendly. But, if weight management is an issue and you are trying to lose body fat, the lower the dietary fat intake the better.

The evils of saturated fat

I'm not going to rehash the things I have said about the evils of dietary fat, and saturated fat in particular. Instead, I'll simply point out that as the intake of saturated fat has increased in this country, so has the incidence of coronary heart disease, and certain forms of cancer (colon, breast and prostate). The average American consumes approximately 15 percent of their calories as saturated fat — that's about 50 pounds per year. Those following a silly high-fat diet consume considerably more.

If you are losing weight while consuming all this saturated fat, what's happening to your health? For that answer, let's consult the lumberjacks of northern Finland. They represent a group of lean and mean hard-working men who on the outside look about as healthy as one can be. They work long hours and have a high level of fitness and muscular endurance. In addition, they follow a high-fat diet, similar to the diet many Americans have foolishly adopted, with most of their fat coming from animal products, and dairy products in particular. Are they truly healthy? Sorry. These men are notorious for dying very early (in their forties and fifties) of heart disease, in spite of their hours of vigorous, daily physical exercise. The reason? A major factor is believed to be their high intake of dietary saturated fat.

To make matters worse, high-fat diets are low in fiber, and lack many vitamins, minerals and phytochemicals essential to health. The lack of fiber and the high intake of animal products substantially increase the risk of colon cancer and other problems.

The Glycemic Index

Several new low carb diet plans are based upon the Glycemic Index (GI). The GI is nothing new, and has been around a long time. It's a measurement of how the foods you eat affect your blood sugar level (which reflects your insulin response). Pure glucose is used as a comparison. Glucose is assigned a score of 100. The closer a food comes to triggering a similar insulin response as glucose the higher the score for that food.

From all that was discussed above, you now know that it's unhealthy to have a huge insulin response to what you eat. Thus, a low GI score is desirable. Authors of diets which depend upon the GI have identified high-responding foods (foods with a high GI) and told readers to avoid them. Conversely, low responding foods are encouraged.

Conceptually, this is not a bad idea. Anything you can do to keep your insulin response down is positive. The problem is, the GI is not necessarily an accurate assessment when foods are combined, as they normally are in everyday life, rather than eaten in isolation. There may be an interaction of starch and protein in food, for example, which alters the glycemic response. The amount and kind of fat, sugar, and fiber in foods also can be an influence

Notwithstanding these technical considerations, it's a good idea to avoid as much as possible foods which drive up your insulin levels. Here are some culprits that may surprise you: corn flakes, carrots, potatoes, maltose (the sugar in beer and malt products), honey, bread, millet, rice (white). Culprits with a moderate GI rating include: rice (brown), muesli, shredded wheat cereal, bananas, raisins, candy bars, spaghetti, sweet corn, bran cereals, biscuits (oatmeal, water, tea), peas, yams, table sugar, potato chips, navy beans, oranges and orange juice. Low rating foods include: soybeans, peanuts, kidney beans, lentils, butter beans, black-eyed peas, chickpeas, apples, ice cream, skim milk, yogurt, tomato soup.

When possible, it's best to avoid foods rated high and moderately high on the GI. Foods with a high GI taken as a snack can create an insulin rebound effect, which results in a very low blood sugar (hypoglycemia) not long after ingestion. The exception would be athletes who take in a high rating GI food for a quick sugar boost during workouts or competition. Such foods taken immediately after a workout can help accelerate restoring the glycogen stores.

Who will you believe?

Thankfully, most people who adopt a high-fat diet abandon it before it can do too much damage. I suspect one of two things happens. Either there are bad effects that are felt immediately. Or, there is weight loss plus all the seemingly good things that are supposed to happen, but deep inside there is a small voice crying out to stop, because things aren't what they seem to be when you go below the surface. Whatever the reason, welcome back to sanity.

For those who blindly cling to the false promise of the high-fat gurus, please be informed that if you hang on too long, you may be sacrificing your future in the process. The bad results may not show up for decades, but odds are excellent that, like termites, the bad effects will become evident at some point.

Confusing, isn't it? Sorry about that. But surely you can see that eating sausage and bacon and cheeseburgers and claiming health benefits in the process is just a little too much for the thinking individual to swallow, despite the quick loss of a bunch of weight. It's simply too good to be true.

So, who are you going to believe? Me, or those who encourage you to consume all the saturated fat your heart desires? Their message is more appealing, I understand. But so is the message of the crack dealer to the crack addict. In deciding who to believe, please ask yourself what I and my conscientious colleagues have to gain by encouraging you to following a healthy lifestyle, versus what others have to gain by telling you the opposite.

The bottom line

Following a high-fat diet is much like bringing in a box full of cockroaches to eat the eggs of flies, and thus solve your fly problem. Indeed, it will work in the short run, and you will rid your house of flies. And in the process you will happily proclaim the brilliance of your actions to all within earshot. But eventually, when the cockroaches take over, your plan won't seem so brilliant. Welcoming huge amounts of saturated fat into your body to replace the sugar may seem like it's working in the short run, but eventually, there is a big price to pay.

The bottom line is, as always — there is no magic bullet, no short cut, no elixir that will save you from yourself. If you want to lose body fat, keep it off, and meaningfully improve your health, you must make reasonable choices along the way.

8. IF HIGH-FAT DIETS ARE BAD FOR YOU, WHY DOES CHOLESTEROL DROP?

In order to explain how it's possible for your cholesterol level to drop on a high-fat diet, while at the same time increasing your risk of heart disease, I'll have to take you a bit deeper into the details about cholesterol. Here goes.

Cholesterol is transported in conglomerates called lipoproteins. These lipoproteins contain many components, including proteins, cholesterol, triglycerides and other forms of fat. The lipoproteins vary greatly in composition, and they are named according to the density of the proteins in the mix. HDL is high-density lipoprotein, LDL is low-density lipoprotein, and VLDL is very-low-density lipoprotein.

Lipoproteins are manufactured in the liver, then released into the blood and transported to the cells of the body where they are used in many ways, such as to help build new cell walls, and contribute to the production of hormones, etc. LDL is the key transporter of cholesterol away from the liver. The problem is, along the delivery route, if the walls of the arteries have been damaged, the LDL may detour into the artery wall, thus contributing to the clogging process (atherosclerosis).

HDL, on the other hand, roams the bloodstream looking for cholesterol that has taken a detour into the artery wall. When it spots newly deposited cholesterol, it grabs it and takes it back to the liver where it can be recycled. But there's usually a lot more depositing going on by LDL than there is removal by HDL, which means the clogging process is progressing.

In a nutshell, then, when it comes to atherosclerosis, HDL are the good guys, LDL are the bad guys. What about VLDL? VLDL is not a key factor when it comes to atherosclerosis. Keep this in mind.

The heart of the matter

When you are obese you probably are insulin-resistant, and the worst thing you can do is load up on sugary foods. The sugar cannot easily enter the cells, even with the help of insulin, so your body produces great quantities of insulin to force the sugar into the cells. This high level of insulin increases the amount of fat (triglycerides) in your blood. Ironically, your triglycerides could be higher on a low-fat, high-sugar diet than with a high-fat diet.

Drop your intake of sugar and your insulin level drops dramatically. An outcome is a drop in the amount of fat (triglycerides) in your blood. This leads to a drop in your serum cholesterol for two reasons. One, VLDL levels tend to be very high in those who have lots of insulin in their system. This contributes to a higher total serum cholesterol. Two, VLDL carries lots of triglycerides as a major component (as much as 70 percent) of the lipoprotein mass. So when you reduce triglycerides, you reduce VLDL, which causes a reduction in serum cholesterol.

Unfortunately, when reducing insulin, there is little or no positive effect to reduce LDL, because LDL has a considerably smaller triglyceride component (only 5 to 10 percent). What's more, eating fatty sludge increases the LDL, the truly bad guys in the system and makes them even nastier.

As you can see, lowering your serum cholesterol by lowering VLDL does not reduce the risk of heart disease, because VLDL is not a key player in atherosclerosis. On the contrary, if, on a high-fat diet, your VLDL drops substantially, but your LDL increases, you are actually increasing your risk of heart disease, despite having a lower overall cholesterol level.

It's complicated, I know. But, because there are so many

people victimizing themselves while believing good things are happening to them, it's necessary to trudge ponderously through the facts. Unfortunately, you won't get this kind of information from those who are hooking you on these plans. On the contrary, they want you to believe in fairy tales and they are counting on the fact that you will never make the effort to look behind the curtain and see who the Wizard of Oz really is.

The solution

First, reduce your insulin level. This is a must. You can do this by eating carefully. When you eat fat, stay away from saturated fat in favor of mono-unsaturated fat (olive oil, peanut oil) which doesn't contribute to an increase in LDL. Olive oil is a big part of the healthful Mediterranean diet, which is healthy because even though it has a moderately high fat component, little of the fat is saturated. Also, consume complex carbohydrates — vegetables (especially soy products), legumes, beans and whole grains. These healthy foods also help keep the insulin concentration *and* the LDL down.

The bottom line

High-fat diets pretend to be helpful. One thing they brag about is making you healthier by lowering your cholesterol. Now you know why this is a bogus claim. High-fat diets are about as helpful as the fox who generously agrees to watch the hen house. Take the fox in and there will be a huge price to pay.

9. HOW LOW IN FAT SHOULD A LOW-FAT DIET BE?

Several years ago, a panel of distinguished nutritional scientists was charged with formulating dietary guidelines for promoting the health of Americans. They examined the evidence in great detail, and after careful deliberation, the panel recommended a diet of only 20 percent fat or less.

But when the recommendation was presented to the powers-that-be, it was rejected. The public won't buy it, the scientists were told. It's too restrictive. So a much higher guideline was adopted — not on the basis of the scientific evidence, but on an assumption about what the public would accept.

In fairness to the powers-that-be, they were probably correct. Recommending that Americans cut their fat intake virtually in half would have been a huge pill to swallow. But at least a legitimate guideline would have been established. As it is, adoption of the 30 percent guideline has caused confusion and harm to the low-fat health promotion movement in at least four important ways.

First, whether intended or not, the public views the 30 percent guideline as optimal. This means that if my fat intake is, say, 34 percent, it's only 4 percent away from the optimal level. Hey, no problem! Nobody's perfect. Obviously, 30 percent is much too high to serve as a reference point.

Second, millions of people who desperately need to lower their fat intake substantially are affected by this guideline. The 30 percent guideline has been adopted by the American Heart Association, the American Diabetes Association, and the American Cancer Society.

Third, many scientists use the 30 percent guideline in their research to determine the effects of a "healthy low-fat diet" on breast cancer and other diseases. Not surprisingly, results of such studies have shown little impact. The appropriate conclusion from such studies should be that the guideline is not very effective. Instead, many have concluded that: "The data do not support lowering the fat content of the diet as a means to preventing disease."

This is a tremendously important misinterpretation, one that is exploited by medical professionals who oppose preventive health measures in favor of drugs, surgery and other fix-it approaches. It's like giving a poverty-stricken family a tax cut as an experiment to see if it will improve their standard of living. It won't, of course, and for obvious reasons. Even so, if you oppose helping poor people, you could use the results of this experiment to conclude that helping poor people doesn't change their standard of living, so why bother?

Fourth, the 30 percent guideline has become a smoke screen for special interests. Producers of fatty foods hide behind the fact that you can piece together a diet that is 30 percent fat by counterbalancing their products with low-fat items. You can, for example, eat sausage if you combine it with several pounds of bean sprouts, giving you an "average" fat content of 30 percent.

Thankfully, there is a strong movement to "redefine" the 30 percent guideline. As a face-saving measure, proponents are now saying that a diet containing 30 percent fat is "transitional." To be healthy, in other words, first drop your fat content to 30 percent, but don't stop there.

Lessons from the Chinese

Despite propaganda from special interests, there is no getting around the wisdom of eating less fat. Medical evidence strongly supports lowering fat intake to no more than 20 percent of total calories. At this level, atherosclerosis (clogging of the arteries) is arrested and a host of other health-enhancing changes occur, including the loss of body fat.

Body fat is reduced even when you eat more food. The Chinese are a perfect example. They load up on carbohydrates, mostly complex carbs in the form of rice and vegetables, and they stay slender. In fact, the average Chinese consumes more calories than the average American but is 25 percent leaner.

Sounds impossible, doesn't it? But it can happen. Eating fat makes you fat; eating good, complex carbohydrates keeps you lean. The Chinese eat little red meat — the leading source of dietary fat in the U.S. — and only 7 percent of their protein comes from animals. Americans consume 33 percent more protein than the Chinese, and 70 percent of our protein comes from animals.

Maybe the Chinese are lean and healthy because they get more exercise than we do. Maybe their lower incidence of heart disease and cancer has nothing to do with fat intake.

Sorry, diehards. True, the Chinese are more physically active than we are. But their leanness and greater health are not due to excessive exercise. For proof, consider the medical studies on the lumberjacks in Finland. These guys get an incredible amount of high-intensity exercise, all day long. Yet they often die at a young age from heart disease. The reason? Their diet— remarkably high in fat, loaded with cheese and other fatty dairy products.

Maybe the Chinese are lean and healthy simply because they are Chinese. Sorry again. When people from other cultures, including the Chinese, come to this country and become Americanized — eating the way we eat — they get fatter, their health profile plummets, and their risk of heart disease and cancer skyrockets.

Can you go too low?

If eating a diet that is no more than 20 percent fat is good for your health, are there even more benefits to be accrued from lowering fat intake to 10 percent? The answer is yes. Dean Ornish, M.D., made medical history with his discovery that a vegan diet that contains only 10 percent of calories from fat combined with other healthful habits (mild exercise, stress management and meditation, group support, etc.), can *reverse* atherosclerosis (clogging of the arteries). Nathan Pritikin's plan for healthful living also advocates a 10 percent fat diet. The Pritikin approach claims remarkable transformations among people on their plan.

Can you go lower than 10 percent? Yes, but you need to be careful. Your body requires some fat on a daily basis, about 3 percent of total calories. The fat must be in the form of linoleic and linolenic acids — polyunsaturated fats.

If you don't get adequate dietary fat, problems can arise. The skin becomes reddened and irritated, infections and dehydration are likely, and liver abnormalities can result. But don't worry. The chances of not getting enough fat in your diet are extraordinarily slim.

A note to those with insulin resistance and diabetes. You need to sit down with a trained diabetes educator or a dietitian and map out a sound dietary strategy. You probably won't be able to follow a diet that is as low in fat as I'm recommending above. Rather, you likely will have to trade off some fat intake for reduced carbs. That's okay, as long as you stay away from saturated fat, and lean toward monounsaturated fat from sources like olive oil.

The bottom line
Reducing the fat in your diet pays huge dividends. If you eat like a typical American, you have a long way to go to get down to a healthy level of fat intake. A good place to start is the guideline of 30 percent fat. But this is only a start, and your ultimate goal should be to get below 20 percent, and the lower the better. Regardless of your total dietary fat intake, reduce your *saturated* fat intake to as near zero as possible.

11. WEIGHT GAIN WHEN YOU QUIT SMOKING

When you quit smoking, you often exchange one health problem for another. You lose the impact of smoking in exchange for a substantial gain in body weight. But make no mistake about it, it's still a good trade to make as the health implications of 20 extra pounds are minor compared with the devastation caused by inhaling cigarette smoke. For that reason I urge you, despite the fear of bulking up, to go for it. And, for those in the throws of gaining weight after quitting, I strongly encourage you to ride it out, rather than returning to the smoking ranks.

Why do those who quit smoking tend to gain weight, and why does the weight seem to come on so quickly? Research points to two factors. One is obvious. When you quit smoking you lose the oral appeasement factor and may eat more to compensate. You are used to having something in your mouth, in other words, and food becomes a substitute for cigarettes. This has been demonstrated among former smokers. Part of the reason why ex-smokers eat more is they are confused. As a smoker, when a meal is over it is typical to light up, thus indicating symbolically that eating is over. But without the cigarette in hand to provide this signal, eating may continue.

Fidgeting and snacking also tend to increase, as ex-smokers crave the calming effect they believe smoking provides. Actually, smoking does not calm you; it agitates you. But when you are used to having a cigarette at regular intervals, you become hyper-agitated when you don't get it, and the only thing that seems to calm you down is finally taking a smoke.

Another contributor to weight gain is loss of the hyped metabolism you get from nicotine. Nicotine from cigarette smoke can account for about a 5 percent boost in metabolism throughout the day. Although this doesn't sound like much, it is when extended over a prolonged period of time. When smokers have this effect going for them, it enables them to eat more without gaining weight. In fact, on average, cigarette smokers consume more calories, and yet are lighter in body weight and leaner (less body fat) than non-smokers.

Eating more has been shown to contribute to approximately 70 percent of the weight that is gained with smoking cessation, and the remaining 30 percent is attributed to the loss of nicotine's boost to the metabolism. There may be something else at work, too, because the weight that is gained is so rapid. Perhaps there is a metabolic rebound factor, and the body's metabolism drops substantially more when you quit (at least temporarily) than the 5 percent boost it has experienced from nicotine.

Some researchers speculate that when a smoker quits smoking, their body thrusts its weight upward to where it would have been had they never smoked, given the number of excess calories they have been consuming daily for years. Interesting idea, but hard to prove scientifically. Regardless, we know the degree of weight gain in ex-smokers seems to outstrip the increased caloric intake which might dictate a gain of approximately 5 pounds in the average person, but adds up to two or three times that amount in smokers.

Weight gain is a huge problem for ex-smokers, and is a common reason for failure to stay away from cigarettes. Often, a smoker will conquer the habit only to gain 20 pounds or more with no let up in sight. In disgust, they return to smoking, because it seems to be the only way to halt weight gain. This is typical in women, especially.

Take precautions before quitting

If you are going to quit smoking, plan ahead. The best way to prepare is to assume you have already quit and must take steps to cope with the changes in your metabolism and your desire to eat more. With this in mind, prior to quitting, start an exercise program and a low-fat and low-sugar diet and create a negative caloric balance (taking in fewer calories per day than you expend). When these new habits are well established, you are ready to quit.

Take your time and don't be in a hurry. The reason is, beginning a new habit requires at least one month, and it takes another month or so for it to really take hold. Ideally, you will know your negative caloric balance is working if you lose about one pound per week. Get into this mode and stay there until you lose in the neighborhood of eight pounds. At that point, you should be able to quit with minimal consequences.

The bottom line

Without question, quitting cigarette smoking is the single most effective thing you can do to improve your health. It's not easy, and there are complications, like weight gain. But, regardless of what happens, it's better than the alternative of continuing to smoke cigarettes. Good luck.

11. SEVERAL SMALL MEALS THROUGHOUT THE DAY IS BEST

I often have advocated the concept of grazing — consuming frequent small meals rather than one or two huge meals throughout the day. In response, many readers have stated that they would eat more and become fatter on such a regimen. Not true, if you eat the right things. Let me explain.

To be sure, if you consumed a typical American diet loaded with fatty calories and sugar, and you ate smaller meals more often, chances are good you would gain weight. The reason is, dietary fat is so concentrated that if you made up your mind to eat more often, you probably wouldn't be aware that in doing so you would be taking in a lot more calories than you would by restricting yourself to fewer larger meals.

When you sneak down to the vending machine and gobble a candy bar and a small bag of chips, for example, you don't perceive this as a "meal," because there isn't much to it. But you would have consumed a whopping 500-600 calories (kcals) — that's a bunch, and it could account for as much as 30 percent or more of your daily caloric needs. Imagine doing this three or four times a day, combined with, say, two somewhat larger meals. You'd balloon up in no time.

If, on the other hand, you were able to eat exactly the same number of calories and the same amount of fat (regardless of whether it was a healthy amount or not), and the same amount of sugar, and you were able to spread this over six meals instead of three, you would be helping your body fight the battle of the bulge. And if you lowered the fat content of your diet in favor of complex carbohydrates, you would find that eating several smaller meals would be a great advantage. Here's why.

After eating, food is digested and the sugar in food quickly enters the bloodstream. In response to the sugar, the body releases a hormone, insulin. Insulin escorts sugar into cells. It also helps promote fat storage by stimulating fat cells in the body to take up fat that also is entering the blood stream during digestion.

The amount of insulin that is released is dictated not only by the amount of sugar entering the blood, but also by the size of the meal. The larger the meal, the greater the amount of insulin released. This means that during large meals that are loaded with fat and sugar, you are putting yourself in the position of maximizing your potential for storing body fat. Smaller meals containing less dietary fat and sugar, on the other hand, would have a dramatically different effect on the body (because of a dampened insulin response) and the result over time would be less fat storage.

The blood sugar roller coaster

Beyond storing body fat, there is another issue. How you feel throughout the day is dictated at least in part by the stability of your blood sugar concentration. When you awaken, your blood sugar level is low due to the overnight fast. That's why the first meal of the day is called the "break-fast." If you eat a doughnut and a cup of coffee, a splurge of sugar charges into the system, creating a huge insulin release. Insulin moves the sugar into the cells quickly, lowing the concentration of sugar in your blood. Thus, in a short period of time you would have gone from a high concentration of blood sugar (hyperglycemia) to a very low concentration (hypoglycemia). When blood sugar drops, you lose energy and become listless and possibly drowsy. This inspires you to grab another cup of coffee or a candy bar in order to spike your blood sugar back up again. But the big insulin response that follows pulls the sugar back down again, and the cycle repeats itself throughout the day.

Alternating periods of high and low blood sugar exhausts the body and makes you feel lousy. It's no wonder that by the end of the day the only thing you want to do is crawl into your recliner and click on the TV. Sound familiar? It should. This is exactly how most Americans drag themselves through the day.

It's time for a change. The perfect solution to sustaining a stable blood sugar level is to replenish the amount of dietary sugar available to the body through the frequent intake (small meals) of complex carbohydrates — vegetables, legumes (various types of beans), fruits and grains. Complex carbs digest more slowly than "simple" carbs (candies, soft drinks, etc.), and therefore you get more of a "time release" effect. The sugar enters the system gradually, rather than in a splurge. And because sugar is entering gradually, there is not a huge insulin response to remove the sugar quickly from the bloodstream. Eating smaller meals also contributes to a lessened insulin release.

The size of your stomach

The size of your stomach can influence how easily you are satisfied after a meal, and therefore it can influence how much food you consume at one sitting. A stomach that is stretched has a large capacity for food, which means you can consume a great deal before you begin to get a feeling of being full. A smaller stomach, on the other hand, will reach the full point more quickly, which will inspire you to quit eating sooner.

In the past, there have been diets which emphasize strategies for creating a sense of fullness in your stomach without having to load it with food. The "water" diet, for example, emphasizes the importance of partially filling your stomach with one or two glasses of water prior to eating. Then, when you eat you will naturally eat less, because you will reach the feeling of being full faster.

This approach is somewhat helpful but it is not the complete answer to losing weight and keeping it off. In our present society eating too much at one sitting often is not the major reason for gaining weight. Snacking on high-fat sludge throughout the day and especially while watching TV in the evening is a big factor. And because you are snacking, you rarely reach the point of having a bulging stomach and feeling full.

It is possible to shrink your stomach. Exercise has no effect, however, because exercise can influence only the muscles which protect the abdominal area, and there is no effect on the stomach itself. The best way to shrink your stomach is to eat smaller meals. Recent research suggests that you can shrink your stomach to three-quarters of its present size in a matter of only about four weeks by simply eating less food at one sitting. Unfortunately, the opposite is true as well; you can expand the size of your stomach in only a few weeks. But to go in either direction, you have to be consistent. Skipping a few meals won't shrink your stomach, and neither will eating like a rampaging warthog for a day expand it.

Given this information, it should be apparent that the worst thing you can do is to skip meals throughout the day and then really load up at night — a typical approach for many Americans. Eating one large meal a day helps keep your stomach stretched, which creates the need to consume massive quantities of food in order to feel full. A stretched stomach also encourages feelings of hunger throughout the day which may inspire too many trips to vending machines for fatty goodies. As if that's not bad enough, consuming one huge meal also causes a huge insulin response which promotes fat storage.

To combat obesity, some people have had their stomachs stapled. This greatly reduces the size of the stomach, and you would think it would be an effective weight loss mechanism. It can be for a while, especially for those who have had the habit of regularly consuming very large high-fat and high-sugar meals. But soon, those with stapled stomachs form a new habit of snacking constantly throughout the day in order to compensate for their inability to consume large quantities of food at one time. They graze, in other words. But because they are not willing to change their diet (if they were, they would not have resorted to stapling), they are grazing on high-fat and high-sugar items, which means their caloric intake may be greater than before the stapling and they get fatter rather than thinner.

The bottom line

The quantity of food you consume throughout the day is important in weight management. But the way you consume it also is important and may help explain why some are obese even though they don't necessarily consume more calories and dietary fat than their thinner counterparts. When planning your meals, take into consideration the fact that a given number of calories (and fat grams) is best consumed over several smaller daily meals rather than a few larger ones.

13. FAKE SUGAR AND FAKE FAT — WHY AREN'T THEY WORKING?

I remember when aspartame (Nutrasweet) was introduced to this country and was immediately hailed as the cure for obesity. Instead, despite Nutrasweet products, we have not only continued to get fatter, but also our *rate* of fat gain is increasing — more of us are getting fatter faster. What went wrong?

Artificial sweeteners were supposed to replace sugar in our diet, and thus we would eat less sugar, consume fewer calories, and lose weight in the process. But things didn't work out that way. Americans simply added sweetener products to their diet, which means most of us are eating more now, and consuming more calories, than we did in the years before Nutrasweet came on the scene.

It's funny when you think about it; sweeteners have had a surprising and misleading effect. Some will eat everything in sight, then drink a diet soft drink or use a sugar substitute in their coffee, believing that use of artificial sweeteners somehow negates the huge amount of fat and calories just consumed. They don't really believe this, of course, when asked. But at some deep level, part of them wants to believe it, and they act accordingly when they are not forced to think about it.

Nutritive and non-nutritive sweeteners
There are many different kinds of sweeteners, and lots of confusion. Sweeteners can be grossly broken down into two categories. *Nutritive sweeteners* provide calories, whereas *non-*

nutritive sweeteners don't.

Usually nutritive sweeteners are used to enhance the taste of certain foods. Because they are high in calories, they are not meant as a dietary aid. Examples include corn syrup, corn sweetener, honey, lactose, maltose, molasses, dextrose (glucose), invert sugar, concentrated fruit juice, and, of course, the sugar we are all most familiar with, table sugar (or sucrose). Thus, sugar shows up on the ingredient list on food labels in many forms. If any one of the above appears as the first or second ingredient in a product, or if there are several of these items sprinkled throughout the ingredient list, you know you have a product that is very high in sugar, high in calories, and is best avoided. Unfortunately, such products became the core of many low-fat diets. Because most non-fat and low-fat foods are loaded with sugar and are high in calories, many who experimented with low-fat diets actually increased their caloric intake and gained weight in the process. That's why many low-fat diets have been a miserable failure.

Items such as sorbitol, mannitol and xylitol also are used as nutritive sweeteners. These are sugar alcohols. They provide about half the calories of typical nutritive sugars, because the body absorbs them slowly and incompletely.

Aspartame, Saccharin, Sucralose, etc.

When it comes to sweeteners, most of our emphasis has been on non-nutritive sweeteners, such as aspartame (Nutra-sweet), which is 160 to 220 times sweeter than sugar. Although aspartame contains calories (4 calories per gram), so little of it is needed to sweeten a product that it is considered to be a non-nutritive sweetener. Aspartame is a combination of two amino acids, and there are some who react badly to this combination and suffer from phenylketonuria (PKU — a rare condition). PKU causes a reaction in the nervous system because of an inability to metabolize phenylalanine, one of the two amino acids.

Other than PKU complications, none of the studies to determine if there are allergic reactions, skin or respiratory problems, etc., have reported damaging findings. That's not to say we are completely out of the woods in the long run. Aspartame is added to thousands of foods, and many of us go out of our way to consume a lot of it. What are the implications of taking in so much over the course of a lifetime? No one knows.

The other big non-nutritive sweetener is saccharin (Sweet'N Low), which is 300 times sweeter than sugar. Saccharin has had a rocky ride in the U.S., having been banned in 1977, because studies indicated it may cause cancer in rats. But it was brought back in 1991, and allowed to be used until the year 2002, pending further scientific investigations. The U.S. is a big market, but since saccharin is being used in foods and beverages in more than 80 countries, what we decide here in 2002 won't greatly impact the use of saccharin worldwide.

At present, foods containing saccharin must provide a warning on the label about the potential hazard to health. Saccharin has an advantage over aspartame, because saccharin is heat-stable and can be used in cooked and baked goods.

Sucralose (Splenda) is 600 times sweeter than sugar, but has no calories. It is made from sugar, is heat stable in cooking and baking and is used lots of places in place of sugar (desserts, candy, beverages, tabletop sweetener).

Acesulfame-K (Sunette) is 200 times sweeter than sugar, contains no calories, and is big in soft drinks. It can be used as a tabletop sweetener and in chewing gum, yogurt, candies and desserts. It's heat stable and can be used in cooked and baked goods.

Fake fats

Theoretically, fake fats should be a good bet to reduce obesity. Research indicates that when you consume products which contain fake fat, you are not likely to consume additional fatty foods later. This is opposite to what we have seen with fake sugar products, and it's encouraging. But such research results were obtained in a laboratory setting where test subjects are not constantly challenged by the availability of fatty foods.

There is another problem to consider. When you look at the American diet, most of the fat we consume comes from cooking with fats and oils (which are entirely fat), and from fatty meats and dairy products. Add these up and you have the lion's share of fat in the diet (as much as 90 percent). Fake fat is not used in any of these items, but rather tends to show up in snack foods. Thus, one can easily be misled into thinking they are doing enough for their health by consuming fake fat snacks. But actually, they aren't accomplishing much if they are not reducing their fat intake in other places.

Creating a good fake fat is a major challenge, because fat not only tickles the taste buds (like sugar), it also has a certain feel to it, and that feel is part of the eating experience. Olestra (Olean) has grabbed the spotlight as the most promising fake fat. It has undergone 25 years of testing and is the most thoroughly tested food ever approved by the FDA. Even so, it still has its critics, and many claim it is far from harmless, especially if consumed in large quantities.

Olestra is made from vegetable oils and sugars, offers no calories, and does a good job of duplicating a fatty taste when fried. The potato chips, for example, taste pretty much like the real thing. Olestra is made by attaching a fatty acid to a sugar, and because our bodies have no enzymes to break down this combination, the body can't absorb it. It passes right on through the gut, in other words. Critics say this is a problem because, as it passes on its way, it takes along fat soluble vitamins (A and E). To compensate, Olestra products are fortified with fat-soluble vitamins. Olestra may cause digestive discomfort and diarrhea. But such problems have, as yet, not caused much of a response from the public.

Another popular fake fat is Simplesse, made from egg whites and skim milk. It's creamy and mimics a full-fat taste fairly well. Simplesse is a protein-based fake fat and is used primarily in low-fat cheeses, ice creams and the like. The fact that it falls apart when heated is a problem. So, for low-fat and non-fat baked goods, food producers use a carbohydrate-based fake fat, which combines with water to give foods a thicker and bulkier feel in the mouth, creating the sensation that you are eating fat.

Unfortunately, as was the case with fake sugar, there has not been a trend toward lost weight and reduced obesity in this country following the introduction of fake fats. To be fair, it's too early to tell, but signs aren't pointing in a leaner direction. Perhaps it's because Olestra products are fairly expensive, and the "real thing" can be bought much more cheaply. Or that items such as non-fat yogurt are loaded with sugar, and there is no real reduction in calories. Whatever the reason, there is little proof to indicate that fake fats will give our nation's health a boost.

The bottom line

In our never-ending search for a magic bullet, we have gone down the roads of fake sugar and fake fat. With all their promise and allure, they have yet to provide benefits such as reduced body fatness and improved health profiles. Will we ever get the message that we are responsible for the choices we make and that we cannot always depend on science to bail us out? Maybe. But not soon. And not as long as there are food producers who promise great things that seem too good to be true, and usually are.

Fat blockers

Orlistat (Xenical in the U.S.) has received a tremendous amount of publicity lately as the magic bullet that kills fat. It has been widely tested in Europe and looks promising in many ways. There was a delay in FDA approval pending investigations regarding a potential increased incidence of breast cancer in clinical trial participants, but the manufacturer convinced the FDA that no such link exists.

Here's how it works. When you eat fat it enters the stomach, then is passed along to the small intestines. In order for fat to enter your blood stream each molecule of fat must be broken down into smaller particles which can pass through the intestinal walls. Enzymes, called lipases, break down the fat. This is where

Orlistat comes in. It blocks the effects of the enzymes, preventing breakdown of the fat. The fat continues along, unbroken, through the intestines and is excreted.

Sounds pretty neat, huh? Well, don't get too excited. Here's the downside. Orlistat is available by prescription only. You have to take the drug with meals, and it blocks about 30 percent of the fat you've eaten. And, of course, with any powerful medication there may be side effects. Diarrhea and abdominal cramping have been reported.

What about herbal fat blockers? Anytime a prescription drug comes out that promises to do wonderful things, you can bet there will be a number of herbal knock-offs which can be purchased without prescription and for fewer dollars. Usually such products don't have the same impact as prescription drugs. If they did, they wouldn't be selling over the counter. I can't speak with much authority on this, but my suspicion is that herbal fat blockers won't accomplish much.

Critics of Orlistat worry about the loss of fat-soluble vitamins (A,D,E, and K). The manufacturers recommend taking a daily multi-vitamin.

In clinical trials, patients were shown to lose, on average, about 20 pounds during the first year from the use of Orlistat, and by following a 30 percent fat diet, combined with a reduction of caloric intake of 600 calories per day. Patients sustained the weight loss over the second year. Health profile improved, with a drop in serum total cholesterol and the bad form of cholesterol, LDL. Both systolic and diastolic blood pressures were reduced, and there was a drop in blood sugar and insulin levels.

These results are encouraging, but let's take a closer look. Such changes in the health profile are expected with the loss of body fat. Moreover, a loss of body fat would certainly be expected from cutting caloric intake by 600 calories per day. That's a substantial reduction, accounting for as much as one-third of the caloric intake of most women, and more than one-forth of the intake of most men. The question arises: What are the effects of Orlistat by itself, without the diet? Hard to say.

The biggest problem with this type of drug, even if it were effective, is that most people will not learn to eat better while they're on it. If they were able to eat better, why bother with the drug? Simply eat better and lose weight and improve your health.

Many people will depend on the drug for weight loss, which means they will face the choice of either staying on the drug for the rest of their lives (a horrible thought), or stopping the drug entirely and gaining back everything they lost (a horrible outcome).

The bottom line

As always, our pursuit of the magic bullet is an amusing one. Millions of dollars are being invested to try to create a drug that will help us rid our bodies of the fat we introduce into it eagerly and of our own free will. Doesn't common sense dictate that such efforts are at the wrong end of the pipeline? Of course. But then, it wouldn't be much of a magic bullet if it didn't rescue us from ourselves, would it?

13. HUNGER VERSUS APPETITE

There is an important distinction between hunger and appetite. Hunger is instinctual, driven by the body's physiology. We have to eat to survive, in other words, and the hunger drive can be incredibly powerful.

But hunger does not necessarily drive appetite, because appetite is largely a learned response to food. Here are two examples. Too often in this society, we indulge our appetite even though we are not hungry. Eating a bag of fatty chips while watching Monday Night football is an example. It's what I refer to as "automatic eating" — consuming food simply because it is there. On the other extreme, a too-thin person who is very hungry may have no desire to eat. This could stem from the overwhelming psychological need to stay as thin, or from a negative relationship with food. Either way, it could suggest an eating disorder, and a physician should be consulted.

Whether we eat from hunger or appetite, how do we know we have had enough? This is where satiety enters the picture. Some experts believe the hunger drive is always turned on unless something steps in to turn it off. How does this operate? I'm not sure anyone knows for certain, but many theories exist. One possibility is stretching of the stomach walls. When they are stretched, signals are transmitted to the brain to shut off hunger. This supports the use of stomach staples in the morbidly obese — stapling makes the stomach smaller and thus turn-off signals would be transmitted to the brain faster. But this operation has not been terribly successful in helping the obese lose weight and sustain the loss, because those with stapled stomachs learn to eat continuously rather than indulging in fewer large meals. On the other hand, some research has shown that animals who have had their stomachs removed still get hungry and want to eat, suggesting that stretching the stomach may have little to do with control of eating.

Another possible control mechanism is the level of glucose in the blood. This makes sense, because we need adequate levels of circulating glucose to feed the brain (the only source of fuel used by the brain), and the body will hardly allow the brain to go without fuel. But research has not supported the notion that the concentration of glucose in the blood controls hunger. If glucose is important, perhaps the amount stored in the liver as glycogen is the key. This is because glycogen from the liver is converted back to glucose and released into the blood stream when glucose levels fall.

Another possibility is feedback from cells that store fat in the body. When they are full, there is no feedback to the brain to eat. Still other possibilities include feedback from the gastro-intestinal tract. When food is consumed, signals are sent which tell organs such as the pancreas (which releases insulin) to get ready to help process the food. The same signals may reach the brain, telling it that eating should stop. There has been a great deal of recent research on missing genes that may control such feedback loops. If you don't have such genes, you may have trouble controlling your eating. (See Part I, #19 for more on the "fat gene.")

As if this were not complicated enough, enter the Set-Point Theory. This suggests that the body selects a weight it wants to be and it does everything it can to attain that weight. How and why the body selects a certain weight is open to question. Nevertheless, the set-point may be a powerful influence. For example, research subjects forced to overeat to gain weight will spontaneously reduce their weight by eating less when the forced feeding is stopped. Similarly, when fat is surgically removed from animals, they will create new fat stores to return to their former weight. Smokers are known to be thinner than non-smokers, even though they consume more calories (kcals) daily. There are metabolic factors associated with smoking that may keep the individual at a lower weight than the body wants to be, and this may explain the sudden weight gain that occurs with smoking cessation. This doesn't mean the set-point of the body cannot be altered. But to alter it isn't easy because the body stubbornly clings to a plateau for a prolonged period of time.

Hunger and weight loss

Is it necessary to be hungry in order to lose weight? The answer is no. Being hungry does not mean you are dipping into your stored fat. On the contrary, as you are now aware, there may be many other factors driving your hunger and appetite. Moreover, if you are on a crash diet and consuming only a small amount of food per day, it's possible that eventually you may lose your appetite. We see this in those who go on prolonged fasts. Ironically, under such circumstances, you are tearing down muscle mass and converting the proteins to amino acids and then to a form of glucose to feed the brain. Fat cannot be used in this way, so the fat stores remain relatively intact. This is why crash diets always fail—you don't lose fat, you lose muscle.

Many factors operate to control the amount we eat daily.

Regardless of which factors are most important in controlling the process, you will be much better off not allowing yourself to get ravenously hungry when trying to lose weight. When you do, you set yourself up for binge eating. Moreover, because of the hunger, you won't be selective in what you eat (unfortunately, fast foods and junk foods are likely to be the most readily available source), and your body is poised to maximize fat storage from the incoming food.

Spontaneous versus regulated eating

While it's best not to wait to eat until you are starving, a good case can be made for allowing your appetite to guide you. This, however, can be difficult, because our society subscribes to regulated eating. At noon on the job it's lunchtime, and we have either to eat, or wait until the work day is done. So we eat, whether we are hungry or not. Regulated eating can cause us to over-consume food, because we get used to eating when we are not hungry. We lose innate cues, in other words, and depend more on external events.

If you work in a regimented environment, consider using your mid-morning and/or mid-afternoon breaks as a time to consume a light meal. You can, for example, eat only a little at noon if you are not hungry, then eat a little more on your mid-afternoon break. This helps shift toward more smaller meals throughout the day as discussed earlier. You probably will have to take your own food to work, but this is a great way to control what you eat and how much, regardless of when you eat it. If you are alert, you usually can find ways to make things work.

14. THE 80-20 RULE SAVES THE DAY

Does following a low-fat and low-sugar diet mean you will never again experience the joys of cheesecake or fried chicken? No, of course not. But you may not indulge as often, and more important, you may not want to. You will be eating more food than ever before, you won't be hungry, and you won't be tempted to give into cravings. That's a big item, because when you are hungry you crave old favorites — the kind of things Mom gave you when you were a kid that made you feel all warm and cozy inside.

Those old urges will always be lurking nearby in the shadows, and occasionally it's a good idea to give in to them. I call this "controlled cheating." It allows some flexibility in your diet that breaks through the rigidity imposed by insistence on strict compliance. The problem with such a rigid approach is that it encourages an all-or-nothing mentality, and once the dam breaks, guilt overtakes you and there's no going back.

During your early days of eating properly, before you have fully embraced new habits and a new perspective, you will be tempted by old favorites. That's natural. The more you are tempted and the more you refuse, the greater the temptation will become. That's why I firmly believe that when the feeling is strong, give in to it. It's okay, because progress toward your goals of a lower body fat and an improved health profile will not be slowed appreciably. Obviously you can't do this every day, or even every other day. But when you start eating the right things and feeling good, you won't want to.

In general, the longer you have sustained a good eating pattern, the closer you will be to being satisfied with your weight and your health profile. As you get closer, you can fall off the wagon more often without ill effects. I call this the 80-20 rule. If 80 percent of the time you are eating the right things, ill-advised indulgences 20 percent of the time won't be a major problem. But for the novice who is striving to reach a goal that is far away, you'd better stick to the 90-10 rule, or better yet, the 95-5 rule, which allows only an occasional bad day.

Taming the taste buds
An interesting thing happens to your taste buds when you follow a low-fat, low-sugar diet for a prolonged period of

time. They become keener. On your old fat-based diet, your taste buds are dulled by a constant flow of rich-tasting sludge. Like addicting drugs, you build up a tolerance and you have to increase the sludge quotient in order to get your kicks. That's why rich desserts such as double-fudge brownies with ice cream topped with melted chocolate and whipped cream are so common.

But after eating in a more intelligent way, you will find your taste buds are more easily satisfied. This has two major benefits. Your taste buds will be more satisfied with less fat in foods. And, because your taste buds are more sensitive, the taste sensation will be extraordinary when they do encounter a rich, sugary dessert.

Won't this inspire you to pursue more fatty, sugary delights? Surprisingly, no. Changes in your perspective on eating, plus changes in your gastrointestinal tract, won't allow it. In the old days, you could eat sludge for days on end without feeling the effects. You probably never felt very good anyway—at least not as good as you could have. But when going the low-fat and low-sugar route, you will be used to feeling good, and when you don't, you won't like it. You won't like the way sludge makes you sluggish, causes you to feel overstuffed, and seems to stay forever in your gut. You especially won't like the effects you will feel after eating something greasy.

Eventually, eating right will win you over completely. You will marvel at the way you used to eat and will shake your head and wonder, "Did I really used to eat that stuff?"

Beware of weight gain over the holidays

When you eat properly, will holidays be a drag, watching others stuff themselves to their heart's content while you pick away at celery and carrot sticks? Not at all.

Admittedly, holidays can be tough, and for that reason you don't want to launch a new eating plan as the Thanksgiving to New Year's holiday season approaches. The cravings and fond memories of food-filled family get-togethers will defeat you before you get out of the starting block. Wait until January 2nd. And by the time next year's holiday season rolls around, you will be ready to cope with it.

That's not to say you shouldn't be prudent during the holidays. On the contrary, don't put yourself further behind because of bad choices over a six-week period of festivities.

Here's a plan. It's divided into two parts. There are short-term, damage control strategies, and there is the more meaningful long-term view which can really help solve the problem.

Short-term strategies

First, understand and appreciate that for six weeks you will be tempted beyond reason to eat everything you shouldn't. Pies, cakes, cookies and candies abound, along with fatty meats and cheeses, plus, of course, a variety of beverages such as egg nog, hot chocolate and specialty coffees; the list goes on. These temptations will confront you everywhere you go, and therefore, the best approach is to pretend you are a Boy Scout—Be prepared! Specifically, don't be hungry when you attend a festive event, because the degree to which you indulge will depend largely upon the hunger you take with you. Eat a full meal first, if possible, then just pick at the goodies thrown your way.

Second, be careful not to settle into a pattern of indulging daily over the holidays. The less frequent your indiscretions, the less overall damage you will suffer. A good way to control frequency is to control temptations at home. Of course, you will have lots of goodies on hand when you entertain guests, but otherwise remove temptations from your home. Be careful of leftovers. After entertaining, encourage guests to take home a "doggie bag" filled to the brim.

Third, alternate goodies with "healthies." After eating a cookie, reach for a chunk of broccoli or celery, then go back to another snack. Alternating will allow you to satisfy your desire for goodies while cutting the amount you consume in half. Also, since your taste buds tend to dull after a series of goodies, alternating with a vegetable will, in a sense, clean your palate and get it ready for another surge.

Fourth, after indulging, take a walk. Walking after eating burns more calories (about 15 percent more) than walking on an empty stomach. The exercise also will take fat that is being digested and use it as fuel, rather than allowing it to be stored.

Long-term strategies

Every year, the average American adult gains several pounds over the holiday season. The problem is especially prevalent in northern climates where the days are short and cold, which discourages outdoor physical activities. Then when the weather breaks and days get longer and warmer we become more active outside and the weight begins dropping off. Unfortunately, we rarely lose all the weight we gained and there is generally a net gain of about 1 to 2 pounds each year. We repeat this process annually from the mid-twenties through middle age and accumulate approximately 25 to 30 pounds of additional fat.

This process, called creeping obesity (discussed in Part 1, #1), goes largely unnoticed because it is so gradual. As we get into our sixties and beyond, it appears as if the cycle has stopped, because our body weight plateaus. Unfortunately, it plateaus for the wrong reason. We still gain our annual 1 to 2 pounds of body fat, but we compensate by losing the same amount of muscle mass. We keep getting fatter, in other words, even though our body weight is not climbing.

Knowing that creeping obesity occurs is helpful, because you can take extra steps to be certain to take off all the weight you gained over the holidays. Have a "weigh-in" in early November and record the weight. Then have a "weigh-out" in mid-January and determine the damage. If you gained 5 pounds, be certain you get it all off over the next several months.

The key is expanding your view to include the entire year, not just the holidays. Use the months from January to November to prepare for the next holiday assault. When you do, you will be able to sustain your weight within a desirable zone without sacrificing the joys of celebrating the season.

15. THE NEGLECTED WEIGHT MANAGEMENT TOOL

If you are a typical American, you are always searching for the magic bullet that will help you manage your weight. And, as a typical American, you probably have been disappointed by a number of so-called miracle cures in the past. I don't have a quick miracle for you, but if you take a long-range approach, I have something that's pretty close. It's pumping iron.

How can that be? Pumping iron (also called resistance training or lifting weights) burns only a handful of calories (kcals) per hour, hardly enough to make a dent in the 3500 calories of energy stored in just one pound of fat. By contrast, walking briskly at 4 mph burns about 400 calories per hour, and jogging comfortably at 6 mph burns about 700 calories per hour. Rowing, cycling, cross-country skiing and other well established aerobic exercise burn lots of calories, too, and generally these are the exercises of choice for those who are trying to trim down. Indeed, they should be the core of any program, because there are many benefits to be derived from a daily schedule of aerobic exercise.

But if you don't include vigorous resistance training in your program, you are missing out on an important weight management tool. Resistance training builds muscle. This is important because muscle represents 40 percent or more of your total body weight, and it largely determines your metabolic rate. As we age, we lose muscle mass and as we do our metabolism declines. Conversely, increasing your muscle mass increases your metabolism.

The numbers game

The implications of increasing your metabolism are quite substantial in the long run. Consider, for example, that a typical resting metabolic rate is about 1 calorie (kcal) per minute. For men it will be higher (1.0 - 1.4 calorie/minute), because men in general have larger bodies, and the opposite is true for women (.75 - 1.0 calorie/min). At 1 calorie per minute, you would expend approximately 1440 calories per day. This is the core of your metabolism. Add to this the energy required to digest food, and the energy you expend moving around and exercising, and you can increase your daily caloric expenditure by hundreds of calories.

By bolstering the muscle mass on your body you can increase your resting metabolism. For example, let's assume you worked out vigorously for one year and added several pounds of muscle to your frame. In so doing, you might increase your metabolic rate from 1 calorie per minute to 1.03 calories per minute. Big deal, you say. All that work for a lousy .03 calorie/minute boost. Hardly worth the effort, is it? I think it is. You will be burning that extra .03 calories per minute every minute you are alive. It's programmed into your system, in other words, and there's nothing you have to do to get the benefit. Given a long range view, you would expend an extra 15,768 calories per year. Each pound of fat contains 3500 calories, and this means you could lose 4.5 pounds of body fat simply by boosting your metabolism. It is assumed, of course, that you don't increase your caloric intake by the same amount. But if you did, it's nice to know that you could be eating lots more without gaining weight. You would be providing yourself a nice cushion, and an increased margin of error that could prevent future weight gain.

Aerobic exercise also contributes some nice numbers. Walk daily for 30 minutes and expend 200 calories per session. That's 1,400 calories per week, and 73,000 calories for one year. That adds up to 20.8 pounds of body fat. What happens if you can't walk daily because you get too busy? You lose the aerobic component entirely and probably will gain weight unless you restrict your caloric intake. In contrast, if you work out one day per week you probably will sustain your newly formed muscles quite well. This is the advantage of weight training. It exerts a chronic effect, helping you 24 hours a day. Aerobic exercise exerts an acute effect, boosting your metabolism only while you participate (and for a short while afterwards as you recover).

Obviously, there are advantages to both aerobic exercise

and resistance training, and therefore it's smart to do both. An ideal approach would be to engage in weight training 2 or 3 days a week, and do aerobic exercise on the alternate days.

Women and barbells (dumbbells)

The concept of combining women and barbells (dumbells) is as old as time. Ask most women and they'll tell you they've lived much of their lives with dumbbells, dating them and even marrying them. But when it comes to the other kind of dumbbell, the solid iron kind, women are less familiar, and probably a little intimidated. They view weight training as a male thing, a foreign concept that, if pursued vigorously, will rob them of some femininity.

This is not true, but it's easy to see how this misperception came about. All you have to do is look at competitors in female bodybuilding contests. Many are as muscular as men, some even more so. But these few examples are extreme, and they are the product of years of intense training, and occasionally the use of masculinizing drugs (anabolic steroids).

Let me add another word about female bodybuilding, just to be sure I haven't left the wrong impression. Most female body-builders go about their training without drugs, and their bodies respond beautifully. A prime example would be Linda Hamilton, the actress who starred in the movie *The Terminator*. She is lean, pleasingly muscular, but clearly feminine. This is the goal of most female bodybuilders. Very few aspire to outdo men in muscularity. I must add, however, that in order to become as lean as Linda you would have to combine a very strict diet with weight training.

When women lift weights, they get stronger and develop increased muscle mass. But because they have a limited supply of testosterone in their system (thank goodness), their bodies do not respond to weight training in the same way the male body does. Results are limited, but that's good, because the feminine physique is sustained while muscle is being added. You will not wake up one morning after a tough workout and see Arnold Schwarzenneger's body in the mirror. You couldn't accomplish this even if it were your goal, so you can relax. Also, because women tend to store much of their fat just below the skin (subcutaneous fat), even with added muscle mass there still will be a desirable level of softness in the physique.

It's hard work

I am a strong proponent of moderate exercise, and I encourage finding an exercise that is fun and comfortable, then doing it every day. Vigorous exercise is great, but few Americans (less than 10 percent) engage is such exercise. With this said, I must admit that if you want to add muscle, it takes a lot of hard work. You can't go to the gym and merely go through the motions. You must challenge your muscles and make them do more than they want to. This is because your muscles will resist your efforts to make them grow. They are programmed that way.

Although building new muscle takes considerable effort, holding on to what you have does not. This may be enough for you if you are satisfied with where you are right now. You would be using weight training as a maintenance measure, anticipating the loss of muscle with age if you don't take steps to avoid it. In this case, a gentle workout, going through the motions without pushing the muscles too hard, will be sufficient.

Getting started

Weight training isn't rocket science, but there's a lot to consider. A good way to get started is with the guidance of a personal trainer (PT). A PT will demonstrate the variety of exercises needed for a comprehensive program and how to perform them properly. You also will learn how much weight to use in each exercise, how to breathe when lifting, how long to rest between exercises, how many repetitions ("reps") to perform and how many sets of reps are best, how to progress, etc.

The best place to find a PT is at your local commercial gym or YMCA. If you need motivation, you may want a PT to guide you through every workout. Or, if you are self-motivated, three or four sessions with a PT may be enough. PT's generally charge from $30 to $50 per hour. You can be trained at the gym, or in your home if you have adequate equipment.

Where's the best place to train? That depends on you. Home training offers convenience and privacy. But you have to invest in the equipment and have the space. Training at the gym is nice, because there are others there doing the same thing, and this is stimulating. You also have a wide array of exercise equipment to use which adds variety to your program. But the gym may offer restricted hours, and there is travel time to consider. In my case, I try to get to my gym, Fitness in Middletown, at least once a week. I thoroughly enjoy the mix of members working out there. I see elderly women heaving three pound dumbbells, working out side-by-side with bruisers pumping out reps with 250 pounds in the bench press. Everyone is polite and accommodating, and it's clear that everyone feels welcome. But when I can't get to the gym, I have enough home equipment to do most exercises. It's nice having both options.

The bottom line

Pumping iron is a wonderful activity that will help you manage your weight, and will help you cope with the natural physical deterioration brought on by aging. If you haven't discovered the benefits of weight training, now's the time to explore. You're never too old, but if you are over age 35, check first with your doctor to make certain you have no underlying health problems.

16. SPOT REDUCTION GADGETS — THE BILLION DOLLAR FRAUD

When I log onto my computer to check my e-mail, or tear into a new batch of letters from readers, one thing is certain. I will be asked my opinion of the latest exercise gadget. Throughout the day infomercials on TV tout the extraordinary benefits of the Flab Fighter, the Stomach Stomper, or the Pooch Puncher. Viewers are told how it takes only five minutes a day to remove inches of unwanted flab from the waistline, the hips or the thighs — all in just one month. Success cases are interviewed. They, of course, have bodies like Cindy Crawford and claim that just a short while ago they were fat and sloppy and afraid to appear in public wearing anything that was the least bit revealing. For the guys, there's Rock Biceps who displays his cut-to-ribbons abdominal muscles and swears he never sweats when he exercises on his Tummy Trouncer.

Such ads promise a magic bullet, an elixir, a quick fix for the layers of flab that depress us when we look in the mirror. A little voice deep inside tells us such ads are too good to be true. But we want them to be true, and as we watch the ads we see that hundreds of gadgets are being sold right before our very eyes, and we get the feeling we are the only ones on earth who are not jumping on board. Desperate, we pick up the phone and commit to four painless monthly payments of $39.95 each.

Six weeks later it arrives. Somehow it doesn't look like it did on TV. Indeed, it's nothing but a few pieces of metal piping plugged together, padded, and painted black. It doesn't feel like you thought it would, either. It's flimsy and stiff and doesn't move quite the way it moved on TV. You lie down on the floor and crawl into it and try to make it do something. You tug and pull and finally get it moving, rocking precariously back and forth. You go through the motions for a minute or two, feeling nothing.

You come back later for another workout. Maybe the lack of effect was due to your lack of experience and knowledge. You rock and roll again, this time for five minutes. No effect. The next day you try again. Still nothing. How, you ask yourself, can they justify charging this much for this useless piece of junk?

The answer is air time. Infomercials cost a fortune to produce and broadcast on TV. Very little money goes into product development; the majority of it goes into their very effective marketing plans. You have been had.

An honest effort

Disillusioned, you wish you had your money back. But you are understandably reluctant to take action and go through all the frustration of cashing in on the money-back guarantee, because you've been there before. But you've had enough, and this time you intend to see it through and get your money back. After 87 phone calls you finally get through to a real live person. You explain your dilemma. They listen attentively and say they understand completely. They apologize and then confess a bit of confusion on their part, because you are the first person to complain out of the thousands of satisfied customers. Then they ask you: Did you put forth an honest effort? Did you follow the instructions to the letter and do your workouts daily for one month? They already know the answer. No. Of course you didn't. This is followed by a pep talk.

Feeling a bit guilty, you hang up with the promise that you will fulfill your obligation and use the machine faithfully every day for one month. You also are bolstered from the pep talk and feel confident that when the month is up you will look like Cindy Crawford. A week later you find an excuse for not exercising. In two weeks your list of excuses has grown. After three weeks you quit and take the machine to the attic and toss it on the pile with the other pieces of exercise equipment you've purchased over the years. Someday soon, you vow, you will have a big yard sale and recoup some of your losses.

What if?

But what if you had iron-clad will power, relentless drive and unwavering determination, and you faithfully used your Tushy Toner every day for five years? Would you look like Cindy Crawford? Probably not. If you made no other changes in your life (switching to a healthy low-fat and low-sugar diet, for example), you would still look virtually the same. Here's why.

In order to lose body fat you have to put your body into a *negative caloric balance*. This means you must burn off more calories (kcals) than you take in. When using one of these exercise gadgets for a few minutes daily, you burn precious few calories — perhaps as few as 10-20 in five minutes. Such a ridiculously small caloric expenditure can easily be overwhelmed by a piece of chewing gum, or a few extra bites at the dinner table. What's more, in order to lose only one pound of body fat, you must create a deficit of 3500 calories!

Even if you were able to burn more total calories while using one of these machines, you'd never accomplish your goal. This is the crux of the matter. Exercising your abdominal muscles may strengthen those muscles, but it does absolutely nothing to remove the layer of fat which covers the area. The abdominal muscles, in other words, cannot reach out and grab the fat that covers them and use it as fuel. On the contrary, body fat is mobilized (set free) symmetrically from all over the body during exercise. You may, for example, during sit-ups and crunches (partial sit-ups which exercise the abdominal muscles more effectively) be using fat which has been mobilized from the arms, the back, or the face.

This is a well-established principle in exercise physiology. Put another way, there is no such thing as spot reduction. You cannot pinpoint an area of your anatomy and decide you will selectively lose fat from that area. No amount of sit-ups and crunches will reduce fat from your waistline. No amount of leg extensions will reduce fat from your thighs.

The only bona fide approach

If your goal is a smaller waist, you must create a negative caloric balance. The best way to do this is with a combination of restricted caloric intake and increased caloric output through exercise. When selecting exercises to perform, it's smart to go with those that burn the most calories per minute. These typically are so called locomotor exercises which move the entire body — walking, jogging, swimming, etc. As you create a negative caloric balance, fat will be lost from the entire body, and, of course, eventually fat will be lost from the areas you desire. The exception to this rule is the stubbornness of lower body fat in females, which lags way behind fat loss from other areas of the body. I'll discuss this in more detail in Part II, #6.

Research studies have compared the effects of hundreds of sit-ups per day with a walking/jogging program. The results showed essentially no change in abdominal obesity from the sit-ups over many weeks, compared with a reduction in abdominal obesity associated with walking and jogging. The reason is simple. The sit-ups burned only a handful of calories per day. This is because the abdominal muscles used in sit-ups are quite small and cannot burn many calories no matter how hard they are worked. In contrast, when using the large muscles of the legs, trunk, hips and buttocks during walking and jogging, the number of calories expended is many times greater.

When doing all those sit-ups, it's possible to mold your abdominal muscles into a rock hard mass. But no one will be able to tell, because the layer of fat overlying the muscles will be intact and will hide the hardness of the muscles underneath.

The bottom line

Billions of dollars are spent annually on bogus exercise equipment touted to reduce fatty waistlines and trim flabby thighs. Save yourself money and frustration by accepting the well-established fact that spot reduction is not possible.

17. PREVENT FAT KIDS FROM BECOMING FAT ADULTS BUT DON'T GO TOO FAR

Body fat is stored in crescent-shaped cells called fat cells, which make up adipose tissue (a type of connective tissue). A hot time for fat cell development in the body is during the third trimester of pregnancy. The more the mother eats and the fatter she becomes, the greater the number of fat cells developed in the fetus. Then, during the first year of life, although the number of fat cells remains stable, they grow in size. Things don't change much until about the age of six, when there is both an increase in the number of fat cells and their size.

Sensitive to this dilemma, many parents determined to raise lean and mean offspring cut fat intake, even in newborns. Skim milk is used, as well as other low-fat foods. Taken to the extreme, however, this well-intended strategy can backfire. Newborns are in a dynamic state of growth, and dietary fat and cholesterol are vital to development. Studies have reported that babies deprived of adequate dietary fat and cholesterol demonstrate retarded development.

But don't interpret this as meaning it's best to pack on the pork. Moderation is the key. Don't eat for two when you're pregnant, and don't try to mold your offspring after the Pillsbury Doughboy. Eat sensibly while pregnant and gain weight in accordance with your physician's directions. Gaining more may add additional unwanted fat cells to the developing fetus, while gaining less could cause development problems.

As a rule of thumb, do not worry about restricting fat and cholesterol intake for the first two to three years of life. Mother's milk will take care of nutrient needs, of course. But for those not breast feeding, follow standard, medically-prescribed formulas. To be conservative, after age three, you can cut back gradually on fat intake. If you want to push the envelope a bit, some experts say you can make subtle changes (shifting to 2% milk, for example) at two years of age. Regardless, starting cautiously at an early age could help your youngster avoid obesity later on.

Beware as kids get older

A substantial portion of American children are obese, and the number is growing at an alarming rate. It is estimated that more than 10 percent of four to five year-olds are already obese, as are more than 20 percent of adolescents. This is of great concern to medical professionals, because childhood obesity tends to lead to obesity in adulthood, which contributes to heart disease, diabetes and other serious chronic diseases.

Children at greatest risk for obesity share some common

characteristics. Either or both parents are overweight. The family tends to be on the low end of the socioeconomic scale, with a small number of children, and most foods consumed come principally from high fat and high protein sources. Too often, kids turn to food to provide comfort in the midst of feelings of isolation, family traumas and abuse, parental loss, etc.

Levels of physical activity among children have declined progressively in the past 20 years. Obese children tend to avoid physical activity, and inactive kids are at particularly high risk for obesity. Ironically, often there may be only subtle differences in caloric intake between obese and normal weight children, and as little as 50 extra calories per day can make the difference.

If your children are inactive at home, you can bet they are inactive elsewhere as well (at school, on the playground, etc.). On the other hand, many obese children would like to be active, but they are embarrassed by their weight and prefer to shrink into the background. If your children want to be active, that's half the battle. If not, prepare for a struggle, but all is not lost.

Reduce TV time

Many experts believe that time spent watching TV is the strongest predictor of future obesity. Parents can turn things around, and the place to start is by reducing TV time. Gradually reduce TV watching from an average of six or more hours per day to two hours on weekdays and perhaps an extra hour or two on weekends. This will prevent your children from vegetating in front of the set and will force everyone to make choices based on quality of viewing. Experts suggest that children can respond positively to this restriction if you approach it as a family decision and allow everyone a voice.

Not only does watching TV contribute to a sedentary existence, it greatly influences food choices. A study by researchers at the Center for Science in the Public Interest (CSPI) should prod every parent into action. They monitored five TV stations in the Washington, D.C. area on Saturday morning and found that 60 percent of all commercials were for food, and 96 percent of these commercials were for fatty and sugary fast foods, chips of all kinds, candy, sugary cereals, salty canned foods and the like. Of the 222 commercials observed, just one mentioned eating more fruit and grains. And even that recommendation was in the context of eating a not-so-ideal cereal.

These commercials have a huge impact that runs deep and may last a lifetime, especially when combined with watching Mom and Dad consume grown-up versions of the Saturday morning fare.

Set a good example for exercise

If you reduce TV time, this will create a vacuum in your child's schedule that can be filled nicely with activities. Whatever you do, be positive about physical activity and set a good example. If you don't have a daily physical activity plan, then start one. Emphasize doing fun things together. Select activities of moderate intensity. Heavy exercise tends to be a turnoff to kids, and to obese kids in particular. Start with easy stuff and gradually increase the amount of time involved. This can be a very effective strategy for weight management, because a calorie (kcal) expended walking in the park counts just as much as a calorie expended jogging. In fact, the walking calories may count more in the long run if they are pleasant and welcomed as part of the daily schedule. Set a goal of a minimum of 30 minutes daily, gradually building to one hour or more. It's not necessary that the activity be in one concentrated dose. The hour can be split into several smaller segments (running errands, riding a bicycle, cutting the grass etc.).

If the children are coordinated, determine their possible interest in activities where size can be a positive influence. In softball, for example, a heavier child may be able to hit the ball with power and be an asset to his/her team. Avoid sports where quickness or endurance is a factor (tennis, soccer, etc.). Non-weightbearing activities are helpful. These include cycling and swimming in which the weight is supported (by the cycle or the water) and is not a factor in performance.

When possible, plan family outings around physical

activity. Hiking, cycling, gardening and family chores (raking leaves, washing the car, etc.) on weekends can be the cornerstone of an exercise program.

Now for some common sense advice. Be patient and be wary of a sense of urgency. Indeed, it's important that things change, but they don't have to change overnight. As a rule of thumb, the greater the change attempted, the less likely the change will last. Anticipate some backsliding, and don't overreact. Simply start the process again, until it is established. Be certain to include the children in the planning process. If they have a sense of ownership, they will feel more positive about the program.

Set a good example for eating properly

Children learn what they observe, and their greatest teachers are their parents. That's why it is so important to learn to eat properly and set a good example. If your child is overweight, take corrective steps, but never put your child on a restrictive diet. You probably will get an emotional backlash, and you may interfere with growth and development. Cut back on fat — it's an effective way to reduce calories without reducing the volume of food consumed. Encourage slow eating, and eat all foods at the table, preferably with the entire family gathered for a meal.

Plan ahead. Get fatty and sugary treats out of the house to avoid temptation, and replace then with healthful snacks. Plan snacks into the day's routine. Take the kids along when you shop, and encourage them, within reason, to make input into food selections. Shop after eating to avoid impulse buying. Also invite the kids to help prepare foods. They may be more willing to try new foods if they help fix them. Never eat while watching TV. Instead, emphasize paying attention to what and how you eat. Try to monitor what your kids eat outside the home. If necessary, pack lunches because school cafeteria lunches often are loaded with fat. Finally, never use food to punish or reward.

18. DIET PILLS

A question that pops up regularly is about the benefits of weight loss pills. Those who ask are looking for a shortcut and they probably know better. But still they ask, hoping that this time the latest pill being advertised will really have a lasting effect on helping them lose weight and keeping it off. Sorry.

Appetite killers

Fen-phen, the ultimate appetite killer, was touted as the savior of the American public, and millions jumped on the fen-phen bandwagon. Let's set aside for the moment the health-destroying impact of fen-phen and look at what was really going on. Users took fen-phen and felt satisfied. A chemical (neuro-transmitter) in the brain was boosted which provided a sense of satiety, as if you had just consumed a big meal. What's wrong with that? Plenty.

When you take an artificial pacifier like fen-phen, what has changed? Nothing, other than the addition of a pill to your life. Indeed, you may eat less and lose weight. But what happens when you quit taking the pill? Everything reverses, and the weight comes back. When quizzed about this exact problem, physicians who touted fen-phen and wrote prescriptions for it responded by saying that in order to be successful fen-phen had to be taken for the rest of your life.

Wow! Imagine starting on a medication that you don't really need, then becoming dependent on it forever. That's scary. Even so, millions bought into it even though scientists didn't know what the long-term implications might be. Eventually those long-term implications were discovered when several individuals developed problems with their heart valves. Oops!

Why would you have to stay on pills like fen-phen forever? Because when you are on pills you are not learning to manage your weight. The pill is doing it for you. Logic dictates that when the pill is removed, you immediately revert to your former state and the weight returns. This is why I always ask those who seek my opinion if they intend to take diet pills for the rest of their lives. They always say no. Then I say, why bother? I follow up with this analogy: Diet pills are like buying a stock that you know you cannot sell. In spite of that, you are enticed to buy it, because you are told that in the short run it will appreciate, perhaps doubling in value. And it does. But you can't sell it; you have to stay with it, no matter what. Eventually the market falls, the stock loses all its value and is worthless. What's the point?

Metabolic enhancers

The other major class of bogus pills are those that boost your metabolism. They are stimulants, amphetamines — low grade "speed." You burn more calories throughout the day and in so doing you burn off some weight.

Setting aside the potential health problems associated with chronic use of stimulants, the same scenario repeats itself. You lose weight while you are taking the pills, then when you quit, the weight comes back.

The best everyday example of how a stimulant works, and how it backfires, is nicotine. In general, those who regularly smoke cigarettes are known to be lighter in body weight, even though they consume more calories than non-smokers. This is because nicotine boosts the metabolism. But what happens when they quit smoking? Not only do they gain weight, but the weight that is gained comes on in an amazingly short period of time. Often there is a gain of 20 or more pounds in just a matter of weeks. This occurs even when they watch what they eat and try not to overindulge after quitting smoking. The reason is a metabolic rebound in which the body delights in being able to gain all the pounds it would have gained if you hadn't been taking a stimulant to artificially hype your metabolism.

Ill-logical logic

In defense of the logic advanced above, those who are determined to take diet pills, regardless of what they are told, tell me that while they are on the pill they will teach themselves to eat better. Oh, really? If that's true, and it never is, why bother with the pills in the first place? Why not, I ask, just start eating properly and allow the process to proceed slowly and naturally. When it does, the effects will last and you will lose body fat and keep it off.

Their answer? Doing it without pills will take too long —to which I slap myself in the side of the head and walk away. After reading what I've given you so far, you must see the folly of such twisted logic. Don't allow yourself to be victimized by foolish diet pill schemes. If you succumb, pull out your cash and go for it if you wish. But later on, after you gain back all the weight you lost, remember that "I told you so!"

19. THE "FAT" GENE

Discovery of the so-called "fat gene" has created a storm of interest. Will it lead to a magic bullet drug that will truly offer long-term help to the nearly one-half of adult Americans with weight problems?

Don't hold your breath.

The discovery that was made may not be as significant as the hype would have us believe. That doesn't mean it's not an important discovery. On the contrary, it may be a major breakthrough in genetic research. The problem is, it may offer precious little relief to the overweight masses. Let me explain.

The gene in question is thought to secrete proteins that control satiety—the sense of satisfaction that comes from having consumed enough food. If you have inherited the "correct gene" you get signals from this gene that are sent to the hypothalamus (part of the brain that controls appetite) telling it you have had enough to eat. The incorrect "fat gene" doesn't send this signal, and (it is assumed) you keep right on eating. The solution, then, is to supply a drug that does the job of the faulty gene. Bingo! No more overeating, and no more weight problem.

While this sounds like a good plan, it depends entirely on the assumption that obesity is an organic problem—something wrong with the body's physiology, in other words. This is certainly true in some cases. Hypothyroidism (underactive thyroid) is one example. (See Part I, #20.) But this is a tiny proportion of the total population of obese individuals, and most obesity experts would reject the organic explanation as too simplistic. Indeed, the causes of obesity and contributions to it are many.

People often eat for emotional reasons, and the more emotionally involved they are (bored, depressed, excited), the more they eat. This is true regardless of appetite. People in our society regularly engage in what I refer to as "automatic eating" —eating when you are essentially unconscious of what and how much you are consuming, because your attention is elsewhere. The organic explanation also discounts the impact of food choices. Eating dietary fat makes you fat, whereas eating complex carbohydrates and proteins will assist you in managing your weight. This is true even if you are consuming the same number of calories of each. And don't forget physical activity. It is well documented that the obese are much less active when compared with those in our society of normal weight.

So, instead of hanging around waiting for medical science to fix your weight problem, take steps on your own. The place to start is to be honest with yourself. If you have a weight problem, I can almost guarantee you have never sustained a truly healthy low-fat, low-sugar diet for a prolonged period of time. If you did (and barring a medical condition such as hypothyroidism) you would lose body fat and keep it off. And if you combined such an approach to eating with modest exercise, your degree of weight (body fat) loss would be accelerated.

I'll repeat my standard advice. Get the fat content of your diet down to no more than 15 percent. Avoid simple sugar products. Keep your caloric intake up to at least 1200 for adult females and 1600 for adult males. Increase your physical activity to the equivalent of 300 calories (kcals) per day (approximately a three mile walk). Choose activities that you enjoy and don't worry about producing fitness. Have fun along the way, and you will keep coming back for more.

Throw away your scale and quit worrying about what you weigh. Use your naked image in a full length mirror as your guide. Give it six months and I think you will be surprised to find that: a) It isn't that difficult to lose weight and sustain the loss; b) Because you are eating mostly complex carbohydrates, you are probably eating as much or more food than ever before in your life; and c) You will feel better than you have in years.

Take a shot. What have you got to lose? Lots of body fat, of course!

20. UNDERACTIVE THYROID

A number of factors can contribute to weight gain, including an underactive thyroid. The thyroid gland is important to weight management because the hormones it releases control the rate of your body's metabolism (the rate at which you burn calories). Even a small change in hormone status can impact your body's metabolism, and, as I have shown you in previous chapters, it doesn't take much of a change in metabolism to create weight gain, or weight loss.

Is it possible that the source of your weight problem is in the thyroid gland? That's hard to say. An underactive thyroid may be present in as many as seven million Americans. The most likely people to be afflicted are women over the age of 40. There are signs you can look for, including lack of energy, fatigue, cold hands and feet, and poorly functioning bowels. In addition, your serum cholesterol may climb steadily if you have an underactive thyroid. If you suspect a thyroid problem, consult your doctor.

There are other factors which could be operating to cause weight gain in women. When you pass through menopause and elect to begin hormone replacement therapy, the therapy can often cause weight gain. Another factor is cessation from cigarette smoking. Those who quit smoking usually gain a number of pounds quickly.

It's also possible that weight gain has been more gradual than you suspect. It is common to gain a pound or two of fat each year over a number of years without noticing the accumulating effects. (Remember my earlier discussion of creeping obesity.) Then one day it suddenly occurs to you that you've picked up a bunch of weight and you wrongly assume that it must have happened recently.

The bottom line is, be cautious and check out any potential medical problems. If none exist, take a hard look at your diet and physical activity patterns. Both may need to be overhauled.

21. THE UPS AND DOWNS OF LIQUID MEALS

Like most things in life, there is an up side and a down side to liquid meals in a can. First, the up side.

Liquid meals were developed primarily for frail, poorly nourished and underweight individuals, particularly the elderly who live alone and have irregular eating habits. They are intended to supplement solid food meals and to add nutrients and calories which otherwise would not be ingested. Others who can benefit from liquid meals are those who are thrust into a weight loss situation from, say, cancer and or chemotherapy, or from an illness such as AIDS. Those who have trouble chewing can benefit from taking liquids instead of solid food. All of these uses are legitimate and serve a good cause.

Recently, some liquid meal products have been touted in advertisements as the perfect substitution for regular meals. If you are the typical busy American, don't bother cooking — just pop a can. If this application fits your situation, there is a down side.

Liquid meals are not recommended as a regular substitute for solid meals because liquid meals are not complete and do not meet all your dietary needs. They usually are composed of water, skim milk, sugar, oil, something to thicken the mix, and artificial flavor, and contain from 200 to 360 calories (kcals), 10-15 grams of protein, 10 grams of fat, and 35 grams of carbohydrates. The vitamin and mineral content can supply anywhere from 15 to 50 percent of the RDAs (recommended daily allowances). As you can see, two or three liquid meals a day would provide only several hundred calories (a starvation diet), and would leave you with many nutritional bases to cover—such as fiber and phytonutrients (healthful stuff you get from vegetables, fruits and grains).

When used as a snack, and in addition to your regular meals, a liquid meal can be helpful. Certainly it is more nutritious and better for you than a candy bar or a piece of cake. But be careful. Can you handle the extra dietary fat and calories? In most cases you may be better off grabbing a piece of fruit, a glass of skim milk or a slice of whole grain bread.

An important item to consider is the cost. Liquid meals can cost $2 or more per serving. That's a pretty steep price for what you get — and much of what you are paying for is the convenience. Another consideration is unwanted side effects. Some people report gastro-intestinal distress from liquid meals, but this is not common.

The bottom line is, liquid meals have a place and can be helpful in some situations. But for the average person, dependence on liquid meals as a regular substitute for solid food meals can be a problem.

22. SOME THOUGHTS ON OBESITY

Over the years, I have worked with countless clients who are trying to manage their weight. I have experienced some great successes, some modest successes, some modest failures, and some colossal flops. Regardless of the outcome, I have learned a great deal from each client, and what I've learned tells me that in the past I tended to oversimplify things. The cause of obesity was clear-cut to me then. It was merely an imbalance between caloric intake and caloric output.

While this is essentially true, hammering away on this theme left many people cold. I now realize that their weight management challenge was much more involved, and the factors which underlie the principle cause of caloric imbalance are complex and run deep in the psyche of the sufferer.

I recently finished reading a book entitled *Understanding Obesity—The Five Medical Causes* by Dr. Lance Levy (Firefly Books, Buffalo, NY, 2000). Dr. Levy believes that 90 percent of those with weight problems have "one or more of the following underlying medical conditions: mood disorders, chronic tiredness, chronic pain, chronic gastrointestinal discomfort, or binge eating disorder." This book makes some interesting points. Some I agree with, others I doubt. Still, it provided excellent food for thought.

To be sure, mood is a key player. A friend of mine who knows as much about weight management as I do, suffers greatly from her obesity. Although she knows exactly what to do and why, she betrays her knowledge at every turn. She seems to be a helpless victim of her moods. When she is sad or when someone hurts her feelings, she's off to the bakery for a dozen donuts. Ironically, she does the same thing when she is happy and excited. She confides that on many occasions she has eaten every last donut in the box, hating herself the whole time.

An evolutionary twist

My friend's story is not unique. But in thinking about her and the points made in Dr. Levy's interesting book, I sat back and tried to envision a larger picture regarding obesity and the factors that contribute to it. Is it possible that many of us (the latest statistics tell us that as many as half of adult Americans are overweight) are victims of a cruel evolutionary twist?

Before going on, let me briefly address the notion of evolution. We are constantly in a state of evolution and, as a result, we get better at coping with our environment. This is necessary for survival. But I am not making any kind of statement or taking a stance regarding the ultimate evolutionary argument —Adam and Eve versus the monkey.

Early man had to search hard for food and eating enough was always a challenge. For this reason, storing energy in the form of body fat was a premier concern. Also, as I have stated, having to feed hungry muscle mass was a daunting task. Thus, the body evolved to the point of valuing its body fat and hating its muscle.

Today, of course, eating enough is not a major problem. That's not to say there is no starvation in the world. There is, and we need to devote resources to stamp out world hunger. But for most of us, especially in this country, we get plenty to eat, and for the first time in history, food is not a leading concern of the populace.

Is it possible that those who consume too much food (for whatever reasons) are in the midst of an evolutionary adaptation, made necessary by the fact that food is plentiful? If so, will this ultimately sort itself out according to the survival-of-the-fittest concept, which posits that those with an enhanced ability to store energy as body fat were likely to be the survivors in times of famine and need? Today, this ability is a burden, predisposing them to a host of chronic diseases, including heart disease, cancer, diabetes, etc. From a purely evolutionary perspective, it could be reasoned that fat-prone individuals would die out, taking with them their excessive fat storing tendencies.

In contrast, those who manage their weight more effectively may have the advantage of having already gone (genetically) through this evolutionary change, and in so doing, have reduced their risk of dying of the kinds of chronic diseases that plague the obese.

Compassion

I have no idea whether any of this makes sense. But it does raise the possibility that many of us have a natural advantage when it comes to weight management, whereas others are behind the eight ball and their daily lives are a struggle against what seems perfectly natural to them—striving to store as much energy in the form of body fat as possible.

If this is true, it makes the case that obesity is much more than a mere inability to be prudent and disciplined when it comes to food. Obesity may be as natural to some as leanness is to others, in the same way that being of a particular race, nationality or creed is a natural phenomenon and something to be respected. As such, it's time to rethink our attitudes about obesity.

There is a need for compassion and understanding, caring and support for those who struggle with their weight. Perhaps Dr. Levy is right. Maybe obesity is, in 90 percent of the population, a medical problem with an underlying genetic predisposition. Certainly, recent genome studies point to a genetic cause in many cases. The discovery of genes which control satiety, for example, suggest that those who lack such genes are destined to eat much more than they need. Is the lack of these genes something that in the past gave such individuals a survival advantage, but today creates great risk?

The bottom line

There is much we don't know about obesity, and until we know more, it's incumbent upon us as compassionate human beings to give our obese brothers and sisters the benefit of the doubt. The obese need encouragement and sane strategies that complement their body's physiology. Weight loss and effective weight management are possible for everyone—it's just easier for some.

23. EIGHT PREREQUISITES FOR SUCCESS

By now I hope you are seriously considering some of the common-sense principles I have advanced so far in this book. If so, here's a final briefing on how to proceed and succeed.

• KNOW YOUR ENEMIES

You can't beat your enemies unless you know them and respect them. The general public doesn't understand the hows and whys of weight management, and is, in fact, remarkably naive when it comes to losing weight and keeping it off. The reason is, what seems logical, isn't. It's logical, for example, to work hard and with great intensity when trying to achieve a goal, and to aspire to accomplish as much as possible as quickly as possible. It's logical to assume that when results come in a rush you are being successful, and the faster things go the more successful you are. And, it's logical to assume that once you have achieved a certain amount of success, you can relax, return to things "as usual," and enjoy the results.

Unfortunately, the above logic not only doesn't apply to weight management, it's precisely the reason why, despite great effort, you almost certainly will not succeed. Managing your weight is a singular challenge, unlike others you have faced, and unless you understand this you are bound to fail.

Steep yourself in the knowledge required to be successful. Success is not accidental, it's not coincidental, it's not freaky. It's the product of knowing exactly what to do, how to go about getting it done, and understanding fully why you are doing it. It's about not falling for silly alternatives, plans that are too good to be true, plans that inevitably lead you astray, abandoning you in a blind alley.

That's why I have labored to present the facts to you, to spoon feed you through the process, to enlighten you to the ins and outs — the subtle yet significant strategies you need to employ and the pitfalls you undoubtedly will encounter. That's why, instead of merely telling you "what time it is," I have taken the clock apart and explained in simple, yet detailed, and easy to follow terms, how it works. And I have repeated some of the more important principles to make certain you get it.

Take time to educate yourself. You must. The time you invest will reward you many-fold. Most notably, once educated, you will know how to climb off the merry-go-round, never again wasting your time losing weight, gaining it back, losing it again, gaining it back again. You never again will be at the mercy of snake oil peddlers who promise the stars, yet deliver only misery, self-doubt and profound feelings of failure. You will see them coming. You will know the lack of truth in their message, and you won't be swayed from your path.

In a nutshell, education will set you free.

• NO MAGIC BULLETS

We live in an era of magic bullets. Penicillin, the Salk polio vaccine, cataract laser surgery, plastic hearts, and so on. Modern medicine has inclined us to look for miracle cures for complex problems, and often it delivers. But nowhere is the magic bullet approach a greater failure than in the weight management arena.

There are no magic bullets when it comes to reducing body fatness. The history of flim-flam crash diets has netted some incredible statistics, revealing a level of failure that can only be described as amazing. It's amazing, because when something fails every time, common sense dictates that we try another path, that we quit beating our heads against the same wall. But when it comes to losing weight, common sense is nowhere to be found. We try the same programs (but with different names, different angles, different deceptions) again and again, always with the same results.

How can we be so gullible? Simple. We don't know the facts, and we are purposely mislead. The always new and exciting weight loss programs are presented with a slightly different twist, which makes them appear unique, better, miraculous even. The options seem endless. Cut your intake of carbs, avoid starch. Eat only protein — egg whites and cottage cheese. Eat several grapefruit after each meal to "cancel" the calories you just consumed. Drink a quart of water before eating. Eat only fruit one day, vegetables the next, prime rib the next. Subsist on a brew of cabbage soup. Eat bacon and burgers to your heart's content, loading up on fat. Consume nothing but raw potatoes.

Three liquid meals a day will melt off the flesh.

Examination of the many flim-flam crash diets we've endured over decades reveals a common link. All of them, without exception, slash calories (especially calories from carbohydrates) to a starvation level, virtually guaranteeing rapid weight loss. It doesn't matter whether you are existing on grapefruit or cabbage soup. The key is starving your body. Do that and quick results are assured.

Herein lies a public relations problem that is very difficult to overcome. It's based in the well-established fact that rapid weight loss not only is possible, but also it's easy to accomplish. Flim-flam diets always appear to be successful. At this point, however, you are aware that rapid weight loss comes, of necessity, from muscle and water, with rather little loss of body fat. You also are now aware that the loss of muscle and water will not be tolerated by the body for long, and therefore the weight must come back. But because the allure of rapid weight loss is so strong, regardless of the type of weight that is lost, we fall victim time and again, hoping against hope that this time will be different, this time the weight loss is lasting and for real. No chance.

Why, despite the proven failure rate of flim-flam diets to remove body fat and keep it off, do we keep coming back? There are two major reasons that seduce us every time. First, our society responds to the need to lose weight with a great sense of urgency. Urgency demands instant results, and flim-flam diets deliver. Second, we approach weight loss with totally unrealistic expectations. We have been taught to believe that we are a failure unless we achieve several pounds of weight loss each week. We are encouraged to get on the scale every day and to expect some decline in weight. With flim-flam diets we get it, and that's the problem. We watch the number on the scale slink ever downward, not knowing that the daily decline, combined with our sense of urgency and our unrealistic expectations, unquestionably seals our failure.

We almost never place weight loss in a proper perspective. Instead, we charge out of the gate, determined to remake ourselves in a matter of weeks. Indeed, we lose weight, lots of it, then gain it back and more. Then, of course, we repeat this cycle, unwilling to accept the fact that the faster we lose it the faster it returns and in greater amounts.

The answer? Accept reality. There are no magic bullets for permanent fat loss, no matter how attractive they appear and regardless of physicians or famous actresses who endorse them. Step back, reduce your sense of urgency, lower your expectations, relax, and proceed with a long range plan. The tortoise approach will always beat the hare's when it comes to losing weight.

• CRAFT A NEW SELF PORTRAIT

No, this does not mean you should create in your mind's eye the picture of you as a sleek cover girl, or a biceps model, and cling to it for all it's worth. On the contrary, forget any image that is far removed from where you are at present. Carrying that image around tells you constantly *what you are not*, which, in turn, creates feelings that you are lacking, inferior, wanting. Instead, accept completely who and what you are. Develop a new self portrait of yourself as a confident, positive-thinking individual. Know who you are and what you are about and where you are going. Know that you can accomplish anything you desire. Once you begin to accept your own inner power, anything is possible. Put the horse before the cart. Get things in place, adopt the proper frame of mind, then pursue your desires.

There is no stronger power in the universe than confidence and positive thinking. This is why successful people are successful. I'm not talking about infomercial gurus who make promises that are too good to be true. I'm talking about good, honest, positive feedback. Surround yourself with it. Arm yourself. Use it to your advantage, and when you do you will be amazed at the effects.

• FORGET THE NUMBERS

Our society is driven by numbers. Each of us can be identified by an array of numbers — social security, birthdate, phone, address—and we deal with numbers constantly in daily life. Numbers quantify things, placing them in context and perspective. Numbers are helpful indicators of progress and success. They also can reflect digression and defeat.

Focusing on numbers is a sure way to defeat a sensible weight management program. Peering at the bathroom scale each morning, rejoicing at a lost pound, or grimacing at a gain, is a foolish way to live. Its effects are numbing, paralyzing, and eventually lead to a sense of futility. Don't let numbers rule your life.

The human body is a dynamic organism which changes constantly. At times it retains water. At other times, water is released. This is controlled by a complex interplay of hormones, mineral balance, and other factors. Tracking your water balance daily is a foolish thing to do, especially if you are going to place any importance on what the numbers tell you. "My water level is up today." Damn! "My water is down today." Hooray! What's the point?

Toss the bathroom scale. Forget the numbers. Concentrate on doing the right things and know that good things are happening. Forget about the rate at which they are happening. Watched water never boils. Watched weight never changes fast enough to suit us. It's the need to speed things up that sabotages us when it comes to losing weight, isn't it?

If you are dying to use some numbers in your program, circle a date on your calendar that is six months from today. Know that on that day you will venture onto a bathroom scale, and not before then. If you are doing anything right, anything at all, you will have lost some body fat during that six month period. But what if you've lost only 5 pounds? Should you be upset and feel defeated?

Not at all. When I do workshops, I develop this exact point, waiting for precisely the right moment to present to the group a model of what five pounds of body fat looks like. It's pretty impressive, and invariably everyone there would accept with great enthusiasm the exorcising of the equivalent of that model of ugly fat from their body. Placing in context that peeling off five pounds of body fat is quite an accomplishment, reduces substantially the need to register big number changes on the scale.

So if you absolutely have to set a numerical goal, how about the loss of five pounds in the next six months? Surely you will reach that goal, and you may exceed it. If so, great. If not, know that you are on the right path and are doing quite well.

• PEAKS AND VALLEYS

Those who start a diet almost always do so with an all-or-nothing mentality. They charge ahead with great zeal, thoroughly captured by the insanity of what they are about. Then, after immersing themselves totally, something comes along which interrupts the flow. Perhaps there is the opportunity to take a trip out of town, or maybe the daily grind becomes overwhelming. Whatever. When this happens, the spell is broken and suddenly there is awareness that the punishment and discomfort experienced on the diet is not worth it. The diet is over. And once over, momentum cannot be reclaimed.

This pattern is typical behavior for Americans. We get excited about something, jump into it with both feet, milk it for all it's worth, then bail out and forget the whole thing. Diets and exercise programs are prime examples. Why? Several reasons. They are, as stated previously, entered with a sense of urgency and expectations that are too high. The regimen that is adopted represents too great a change in lifestyle, and the greater the change the less likely it will last. And changes that are adopted are viewed as short-term rather than life-long.

There is a better alternative. If the diet and exercise plan you adopt is reasonable, comfortable, and health-promoting, chances are good you will want to stick with it for the rest of your life. It represents a meaningful lifestyle change, in other words. This is good. But it doesn't necessarily mean you won't have bad days, bad weeks, or even bad months. You will, and when you do, you may cheat on your diet or crash on the couch. That's okay. It will pass, and when it does, pick up the pieces, get back on the wagon, and start again.

Every lifestyle element has peaks and valleys. It comes with the territory. The key is, over the long haul there is a sustained pattern that ultimately leads to success.

• A TIME FOR SELFISHNESS

Often I find that one spouse will pledge to do the right things when it comes to diet and exercise only to have their efforts sabotaged by the other spouse (usually the husband) who won't even think of tasting something that isn't loaded with grease. The well-intentioned one will hang in there for a while, then collapse under the load of trying to adjust their own lifestyle, with all its challenges, combined with a relentless assault from their significant other.

To this I say it's time to be selfish. Selfish? What a terrible thing to say. Not really. If you are going to be successful with the approach I advocate, you must increase your personal status. You must elevate yourself and make yourself a priority. This is not easy, to be sure, especially for those who by nature are loving, giving, and nurturing people. This may be the most difficult challenge you face. Do it anyway. You are worth it.

• VALUE YOUR PERSONAL EXPERIENCE

We humans like to believe we are rugged individualists, and, indeed, some of us are all of the time, and most of us are some of the time. But when it comes to things we don't understand, we are herd-oriented creatures who faithfully follow the pack. We see a preposterous new diet touted on TV with claims that are too good to be true, and we're off to the races. Our friends and neighbors jump on board and before you know it, the nation is in a new diet frenzy that spreads like wildfire. The same is true for new exercise gadgets which promise trim thighs and slim tummies. We buy them in a rush, then abandon them as quickly.

Ironically, in other areas of our life, we learn from our first experience. If we bought swamp land in Florida from a charming telemarketer, we'd never dream of repeating the same mistake. As the saying goes, "good judgement comes from experience, and experience comes from bad judgement." And if a friend, someone you knew and trusted, called to share a hot tip on a great land deal he'd heard about in Tahiti, you would have no trouble telling your friend that your experience has taught you a valuable lesson, and that your answer is, no.

If you are an American, chances are good that you have tried a variety of flim-flam diets. Your experience has taught you they don't work. Trust your experience and don't repeat mistakes of the past. Combine your experience with the new-found knowledge of how weight management issues truly operate and you will forever more be in a position to make good choices that will serve you well. Another saying applies: "Fool me once, shame on you. Fool me twice, shame on me."

• SET PROCESS-ORIENTED GOALS

Self-help gurus emphasize the importance of goal setting. Indeed, in order for the power of positive thinking to work, you have to have your mind set on an outcome, a goal. We are taught to define goals specifically; to establish ways of measuring progress with smaller immediate goals along the way; to not be too outlandish in our quest, but rather to establish ultimately reachable goals. You get the idea. These are good thoughts which can serve you well.

Unfortunately, however, goal setting can be a tyrannical trap which can lead to obsession and irrational behavior. Weight loss is the perfect example. You want to lose 40 pounds. That's the goal. It's specific and can be subdivided into smaller goals — losing 10 pounds the first week, for example, which can be tested and counted as progress. We've all done this. It's the heart of any weight loss plan. It's also the heart of weight loss failure.

How can we get around this trap? Instead of establishing hard and fast "product-oriented" goals that are closely monitored, I suggest first establishing "process-oriented" goals. Establish the goal of doing the right things for a month. Change your diet in ways I recommend and include some physical activity in your daily life. Don't be too ambitious in your approach at first. Instead, concentrate on the process of change, making certain you do something toward your goal each and every day. It takes about a month to establish the beginnings of a new habit, and that's exactly what you are trying to do. At the end of the month, pat yourself on the back and set a new goal of continuing the same course for the next five months.

Periodically, but not too often, check to see how well your *process* orientation is working by assessing the *product*. As stated above, at the six month mark, get on a scale and see what you have produced (in terms of weight loss). If you have accomplished your process-oriented goal, you also invariably will have achieved some production. Embrace the product, no matter how small, as a success. In this way, you will have shifted your attention to doing the right things—toward the means, rather than the end. In this approach, the product becomes incidental.

Concentrating on the means ensures success, especially in the long term, because you can control the means, and no matter how you cut it, the key to success in any venture is control. With the process-oriented approach, you will exert total control over the issues, rather than being controlled by them. You will no longer evaluate your status (and your worth as a human being) on the basis of what you have produced (which often is beyond your control), but rather on how you have approached it—the process (which is entirely under your control). Along the way, results will occur—you will produce a product. But you will have proceeded comfortably and in a manner that is consistent with true lifestyle changes which can be sustained.

If your ultimate goal is to lose 40 pounds, you will get there. Does it matter if it takes a year? Two years? Didn't you take several years putting on those 40 extra pounds? And isn't it true that the faster you take it off the faster it comes back? Taking your time improves the odds that whatever change you have produced will be permanent. Taking your time also allows you to be more relaxed and to enjoy the journey. Speeding things up automatically makes you uncomfortable.

To make this point, envision a journey on foot of many miles. Your goal is to get to your destination. One approach is to take off as fast as you can. With your fast start you cover the first mile quickly and you are bolstered at your fast progress. But such an approach is uncomfortable and you quickly fatigue. Fatigue causes you to concentrate on how much longer you must endure, how much more pain you must experience before you achieve your goal. Soon, of course, the fatigue and pain are too great and you must stop. Usually at this point you abandon your goal as unreachable. You simply can't get there in this way.

Conversely, if you begin walking at a comfortable pace, you can forget about the ultimate destination. You feel good as you move along the path and you find you are enjoying the scenery and the smell of roses along the way. Because you are in no hurry and are actually enjoying the journey, you are surprised when you reach your destination. Your arrival is of secondary importance to the journey itself.

The process-oriented approach removes time pressure and eases the burdens imposed by a workhorse, productivity ethic. By emphasizing the process, you will finally arrive where you want to be. It's inevitable. The best news is this: In progressing toward your goal you will marvel at how comfortable the approach is and how good it feels. Try it. It works.

PART II

FOR WOMEN
(and those who care about them)

INTRODUCTION

PART II is written for women, with emphasis on the daunting challenges women face when it comes to weight management. That's not to say men should avoid this section. On the contrary, in order for women to maximize, internalize and apply the wisdom and insights provided, they will need considerable support from one another and from the men in their lives. In addition, much of what is being directed at women, also applies in some ways to men. This is especially true when considering the contributions we men have made to many of the challenges women face.

The goal of PART II is to stimulate your thinking, and to set you on the right path. Chances are good that most of what you think you know is false, a product of decades of mis-information, flim-flammery and downright deceit. Chances are quite good that if you are a woman you have allowed your self-perception and body image to be molded by others who do not have your interests at heart, and who have much to gain by keeping you dissatisfied and eager to improve. When you are in such a state you are easily influenced, and ultimately you are completely controlled. Try as you may, you believe you never measure up, and no amount of abusive and punitive dieting seems to get the job done. Ever wonder why? I'll discuss this in detail.

Sure, there are fleeting moments of triumph, such as when you finally squeeze into that size 8 dress just in time for your high school reunion. But you know it won't last, because you did crazy things to get there. And sure enough, it doesn't. In no time, the weight is back and you are again defeated and frustrated. But you wait for the next diet scheme to come along. You grab it, only to fail again and again.

Almost every adult American female beyond the age of 30 has battled with her weight to one degree or another. Some are doing the right things and are successful. When they read the words in this section they will be nodding their heads, saying "Yeah, I know that," and, "Yeah, I do that already." Unfortunately, they will be a minority. To the rest, this section will challenge everything you've been taught to believe about yourself, and about how to manage your weight.

For starters, maybe you are doing a whole lot better in the weight management department than you think you are, and maybe you should rethink your need to lose so many pounds. A good first step is to ask yourself if your need to lose weight is for health reasons or purely cosmetic reasons. Do you know the difference, and do you know why the difference is critical to your efforts? I'll tell you.

This is radical stuff, because everything you read in this section is likely to be contrary to what you believe to be true. It's contrary, because it's common sense and it's backed by scientific evidence.

Take a risk and undo your past thinking on weight management. Restructure your philosophy and step into a whole new world. What have you got to lose? Your past efforts have failed miserably, so why cling to them? What do you have to gain? Everything—a new attitude, a refreshing sense of self-acceptance, and a healthy new body you can live with and love.

1. UNCOMMON SENSE: WHAT'S LOVE GOT TO DO WITH IT?

Many spiritual beliefs emphasize the notion that there are two primary forces in our nature — love and fear. Love breeds acceptance, caring and compassion, while fear breeds rejection and hatred. It is natural to hate what we fear. If I fear that those around me won't love me because my body is not acceptable to them, it follows that I, too, will find my body unacceptable and I will hate my body for failing me.

Talk to the average middle-aged woman about weight management and you will hear a story about adversaries. The adversaries are her true self versus the perception of herself. If she is typical, her perception is that her body is unacceptable, and to overcome this she works hard against her body, assaulting it with the punitive approaches advocated in the typical crash diet. With her body under attack, it responds, she gets thinner and she is more acceptable to herself. But always, her body betrays her. Or so she thinks.

Indeed, the weight she lost always comes back, and usually in a rush. But does the fact that the weight always comes back reflect betrayal on the part of her body? No! Her body has not betrayed her at all. On the contrary, her body is protecting her by rejecting the punishment of the crash diet and fighting against it with all its might, knowing that it is harmful to her. Even so, she comes back again to "newer and better" diets which promise much but deliver only heartache, failure, and more self-loathing.

When we operate in a spirit of love, the universe is with us. We are in balance, everything is as it should be, and things work together for the greater good. Life is enjoyable, and life is "lived" each day. That's not to say there is perfection. Not at all. But there is growth and upward movement. When we operate in a spirit of love, the upward movement, while slow, is certain. There also is confidence that we will reach the goal, and therefore there is no need for hurry and worry, and certainly no need for desperate actions. Regarding weight management, I call this the biosynergic (working with the body in a spirit of love) approach.

By contrast, when fear takes over, balance dissolves and everything falls apart. There is a sense of desperation leading to desperate acts, and such acts are the antithesis of love. They are assaults, directed at whomever is responsible for our fear. Often our assaults are outwardly directed—at our boss, the government, the neighbors, etc. But when it comes to weight control, the villain is our body and the assaults are pointed inward. Our body must be brought under control or else. No approach is too extreme. No approach is unjustified.

But try as we might, our bodies resist our efforts. Despite the small sham victories over our bodies that come with short-term desperation approaches, our bodies always bounce back, thumbing their noses at us, making us hate them all the more.

Is it any wonder that our hateful approaches always fail? Of course not. They must. Love always wins over fear. Fear may have the upper hand for brief periods, but love always is victorious in the end.

You have a choice. You can continue battling against your body, assaulting it with hateful actions, or you can turn the tide with love and take the biosynergic approach. Love your body and work with it toward reasonable goals. Goals of health, energy, feeling good, and, yes, looking good. And most important, you can live while you change. You no longer will place yourself in a horrible dark cocoon, hoping that six weeks from now you will emerge with an acceptable body. Instead, you will start from a position of love, working with your body, and you will be amazed at how your body will respond.

Maybe this sounds to you like New Age mumbo jumbo. But think about it in real-life, everyday terms. If you have a puppy and begin training it, which approach do you think would be most effective — hateful assaults on the puppy if it does not immediately comply with your wishes, or love and acceptance when the puppy does something you like? Would you want your son or daughter to play for an emotionally abusive little league coach who berates them for not measuring up? Or would you prefer a loving and caring coach who recognizes small successes and rewards them effusively?

The answer is obvious. Just ask a trainer, a coach, or a teacher; they'll tell you that love and acceptance work miracles, while attacks and assaults result in confusion, fear, disastrous results, and long-term psychological damage.

There are hundreds of examples of how love can get the job done, and how hate fails every time. Watch the effects of a loving compliment and compare them with a cutting criticism. The compliment inspires a smile and a loving gesture in return, while the criticism returns wrath and hatred. Allowing someone to merge in traffic brings a smile and a wave, while competing and beating someone to the spot inspires rage.

Imagine how your poor body feels when it never hears

anything from you but criticism and negativity, and when it comes to weight management, never experiences anything but brutal assaults. Imagine how it feels when you punish it with the latest crash diet. Imagine how it feels when you abandon the crash diet and gorge on all the things that increase your girth, inspiring even more self-hatred. Can you imagine living every day under such circumstances? You'd go mad! You'd probably go deep inside and rarely allow yourself to surface for fear of another assault. Well, in a manner of speaking, our bodies have gone mad. They are braced for the worst and resist every step we take, knowing the outcome in advance, knowing that more hatred is waiting just around the corner.

Time for a change

It's time for a change in our thinking, and that's the purpose of this section. But before getting too deeply into my message, let me emphasize what this section is not. This section is not a self-help cliche, espousing the "accept yourself as you are, even if you are too fat," theme. It does not attempt to glorify obesity, or convince you that carrying too much extra baggage is okay. It's not. Too much fat on your body can be a health problem which must be addressed.

But not all excess fat is unhealthy, and carrying some extra flesh is not necessarily obesity. Research has shown that if you are within approximately 20 percent of your ideal weight, your health is probably not in danger. This means if you weighed 132 pounds in your twenties, and you weigh 158 pounds two decades later, it's probably not a health issue. (But don't take your health for granted. Get check-ups regularly to be certain.)

With this said, the choice to reduce from that 158 pounds is likely to be purely for cosmetic reasons. And if we accept that having some extra flesh is not only natural but attractive, it opens the door to imposing standards that are less harsh. An option is to stay at 158 pounds, or lose a little, down to 150, or even 140, if you must. But you clearly don't have to drive yourself back to the 130's to be acceptable. This approach is not only easier, it will hopefully lead to self-acceptance and a happier lifestyle, which ultimately will be a healthier lifestyle. Let me add that changing to a healthier low-fat and low-sugar diet as presented in the Jack Sprat Low-fat Diet can improve your health profile, whether you lose weight or not.

Taking charge

It's time to release the suppressed majority of women in this country from an unbearable yoke, from the unreasonable ideals thrust upon them by the media, by men, by outsiders who couldn't care less what price they pay to comply. Ironically, women are the only ones who can remove the burden. Women must retake command of their bodies and learn to live in peace with proportions that are natural and comfortable and healthy. The women of this country must unite and scream, "Enough is enough!" It's time to abandon the all-or-nothing approach we've been taught. The "cover girl or bust" philosophy has condemned the women of this country to a life of repeated crash diet failures and deeply ingrained self-loathing.

Is there any chance women can break out of this trap? Yes. An example is the response of women to the fashion industry. Over the years, the fashion industry has dictated what is in style — what is acceptable. Styles generally change every few years, requiring that women revamp their wardrobes to suit, spending lots of cash in the process. Men do some of this, too, but the impact is not nearly as great.

A few years ago, I was heartened to see women rejecting a return to the mini-skirt. Now, don't get me wrong. I think mini-skirts are great. But I hate that a handful of designers in Paris or New York can dictate what women should wear, and I saw this rejection as a major breakthrough. It allowed women to gravitate toward the mini-skirt look if they chose, and it also allowed them to turn their backs on it. Today, it appears that women can wear ankle-length skirts if they like, skirts that run to knee level, or the mini-skirts, and not feel that they are violating some sacred style rule.

The bottom line

Women have come a long way in this society, fighting tooth and nail for the right to vote, the right to receive equal pay for equal work, etc. The time is ripe for another important battle — the battle for women to reclaim their own bodies. It can be done. The solution? Tell men, the media, fashion gurus, and whoever else thinks they have the right to dictate what is best for you, to step aside and mind their own business. Go for it. The prize has incredible implications for leading a more peaceful, joyful and healthy life.

2. FAT VERSUS FULL-FIGURED

As a starting point for changing attitudes, let me define the terms "fat" and "full-figured." I have defined "fat" to mean a state of excess body fatness which endangers health and well-being. I have defined "full-figured", on the other hand, to mean a perfectly healthy state of fleshiness, one that should be accepted and embraced as natural for adult women in our society. Unfortunately, the full-figured look is ostracized at present and a too-thin standard has been substituted in its place. Very few women meet this too-thin standard, but countless numbers pursue it. And in pursuit of it, eventually they boomerang, going from thin to full-figured again, and then upward and onward, ending up fat. Crazy, isn't it?

In our society, fat and full-figured often are confused as the same, and full-figured women who otherwise are doing quite well find themselves constantly jousting at windmills, fighting a battle that is not only not worth fighting, but is entirely unnecessary.

To help make this point, I have coined the term "fool-figured" and defined it to mean the foolish pursuit of a too-thin look—a look that is virtually impossible for the masses. Pursuing it invariably leads to frustration, disappointment, self loathing, and most important, to being "fat."

In reading this section you will confront a choice. You can continue grasping relentlessly for the too-thin, fool-figured look, endangering your health and altering your body's physiology in favor of storing even more fat in the future. You can, in other words, continue to work against your body as if it were your enemy. Or you can embrace yourself in love, seek an achievable middle ground, work toward that goal by working with your body biosynergically, and improve your appearance and health along the way. The wisdom in support of the latter choice is profound and convincing. Unfortunately, today most women choose the former out of ignorance and pressure (real or imagined) from society, and from men in particular.

Sarah

Sarah is a perfect example. (Note: Names have been changed to protect privacy and confidentiality.) When I met 43 year old Sarah she weighed 148 pounds. She was, at 5 feet 3 inches tall, an attractive woman, dressed smartly in business attire. She came to see me because she was dissatisfied with her present condition. I listened as she explained how she had already lost close to 50 pounds. Despite her success, there was clear self-disdain for not having achieved the level of perfection she sought. She was determined to reach 110 pounds (her weight in college), approximately half the weight she had been carrying for years. Preposterous, I thought — at her height and age, a weight of 110 pounds would be nearly impossible to attain without starvation, and clearly impossible to sustain. But she was so motivated, I couldn't rain on her parade. I agreed to assist her in any way I could, hoping that ultimately she would listen to reason, and revamp her goal to a more reachable and sustainable level.

After losing 50 pounds, Sarah's body began to resist her efforts. To this point she had been following the Jack Sprat Low-fat Diet, which included sane eating and ample daily physical activity. It had worked fine for nearly two years, and her efforts represented an almost textbook example of what is possible and how well things can work if approached correctly. But now things were getting tougher and her body wouldn't yield fat as readily as it had.

I told her this was natural and encouraged her to give it more time and that eventually she would get closer to where she wanted to be. Losing body fat, I explained, is not always a linear process; her body may want to stay at a particular weight for a while, adjusting to it. We refer to this as a period of consolidation. Physiologic consolidation periods are natural, and are especially likely to occur as overall fat stores dwindle. I admonished Sarah that her goal of 110 pounds may not be realistic. She didn't want to hear it. She had experienced success and wanted more. She needed more in order to fully accept herself. My pleas not to do anything rash fell on deaf ears.

Later I learned that she had abandoned the common-sense approach she had been using, adopting instead a well-known crash diet that supplied less than half the calories she had been consuming. In the process, she thrust her body into a survival mode, starving herself, and sure enough, the pounds came off. Unfortunately, such a move caused the loss of muscle mass, not fat (as discussed in detail in Part I). In less than two months she achieved her goal of 110 pounds.

She was ecstatic when she came to see me, dressed in a new outfit, and I could detect more than a hint of smugness in her voice. Outwardly, I shared her enthusiasm, congratulating her on her accomplishment. Inwardly, I worried. She had lost her glow. It was replaced by a sunken appearance, the look one takes on when battling a chronic illness. The scale may have told her "congratulations, you have reached your goal." But her body was telling her something quite different. It was telling her how unnatural it felt and how unhealthy it had become. It was telling her that it couldn't survive in this state for long and that things must change drastically and soon.

"What now?" I asked. My question seemed to surprise her. She responded that she was where she wanted to be and that she intended to stay there, no matter what. I knew better, but I kept it to myself. Doing desperate and foolish things to achieve a goal in the near term is one thing, but continuing down the same path for the rest of your life is quite another. I later learned that to reach this unreasonable weight she had often gone without eating for an entire day, then ate, then fasted again. Later, when she had returned to sanity, she admitted to feeling weak and often dizzy during that time, almost as if she were existing outside her body. I knew her approach was extreme, but I had no idea how extreme. She literally was killing herself. Eventually, she drove her body to illness and had to abandon her suicidal approach.

Predictably, it didn't take long before Sarah's weight began to rise, and as it did so did her avoidance of me. Eventually, we met face to face, and when we did it was apparent she was well above the 148 pounds she had carried when we first met.

Another chance encounter months later revealed even greater weight gain. Clearly, she was sprinting back to where she had started. How could this highly intelligent and accomplished woman fall, despite common sense, despite a strong desire and determination, and despite my warnings, into such a predictable trap? Why did she abandon her original strategy that had been working so well? Why couldn't she be satisfied at a more sustainable weight, rather than forcing herself down to a weight that brought catastrophic results?

It was then that I realized that even though my approach to weight loss was scientifically based, filled with common sense, tried and proven, it lacked something when it came to women. It lacked perspective and an understanding of the deeply-rooted nature of weight control and its significance to the female psyche. It lacked appreciation for the totally unrealistic expectations we men impose upon women (and, in turn, women impose upon themselves) and the emotional toll these expectations exact.

I saw something else, too. I saw that when it comes to bodies, women who easily condemn themselves, are loving, forgiving and accepting of others. They accept the plumpness of their man as natural, never questioning how much better he would look by shedding 20 pounds or so, reducing his pot belly, trimming his love handles. This doesn't mean women don't notice. They do, and they appreciate an attractive male figure. But it's not so important as to impose an unrealistic standard on their mate, making him uncomfortable with himself, creating a subtle undercurrent of rejection.

Unfortunately, we men are not so noble. We easily accept our own anthropometric (bodily) imperfections and fully expect others to do the same, but we reject out of hand a less than perfect female physique. We point at the speck in the eye of a woman, while ignoring the log blocking our own field of vision.

The thinness trap

So deep is this negative body image that males in our society, myself included, cannot grasp it. But the more experiences I have, the greater my growth and appreciation. Molly has made a great contribution to me in this regard.

Molly (not her real name), an attractive young woman, visited my office recently seeking advice. She had once weighed 497 pounds and now weighed 180! At 5 feet 10 inches, she looked great, with measurements of 41-28-38. She recounted with good humor what life was like at nearly 500 pounds: Her frequent $15 trips through the McDonald's drive through, for example, in which she ordered two large drinks, hoping those inside would think her massive order was for two; how her small car would lean to one side when she got in the driver's side; and how, eventually, she couldn't get in the car anymore, and broke the seat trying. Despite the humor, it wasn't hard to sense the pain associated with the ridicule and rejection she faced daily from everyone in her life, including her family. Then, after hearing repeated warnings from doctors that she would die if she didn't lose weight, she decided to change. When she did she grabbed her weight problem by the throat and wouldn't let go.

Molly told me she was dissatisfied at her current 180 pounds and was determined to lose another 30 pounds. She wanted my advice on how to proceed, because, in her opinion, she was still too fat. I was astonished. To me, this young woman deserved an award for a singular accomplishment that is far beyond anything achieved by anyone I had ever worked with. Instead, she was dissatisfied with herself, and disappointed with her "failure."

She told me she was exercising hours daily and restricting herself to 1350 calories (kcals) and less than 20 grams of fat per day. She showed me her journals which recorded in detail every morsel of food she consumed and every exercise session she completed in the past six years. I listened and agreed that she was doing everything right. Indeed, the loss of more than 300 pounds attests to the success of her program. But these last 30 pounds were stubborn. Her weight had plateaued, not budging a pound for quite some time.

I had no reasonable suggestions for changing her program. On the contrary, if she hadn't told me she was doing this for the past six years, I would have told her she could never sustain such a Spartan approach.

Instead of helping her revise her program, I encouraged her to invest some of the effort she was putting into exercise and dieting into self examination and self acceptance. She needed to lighten up. She was surprised at my message. She thought I would condemn her for eating too much or not exercising enough.

From the look on her face I could see that Molly was disappointed. She wanted input on how to overhaul her diet and exercise regimen, and it was obvious she stood ready to do anything I advised, no matter how ridiculous it might be. She was ready to do outlandish things, but was not ready to do the sane thing—give up her unrealistic goal. Instead of congratulating herself and valuing her accomplishment, she was lost in the wilderness of a hopelessly negative self image. No amount of effort on my part over the two hours we talked could budge her. She would politely nod her head as I spoke, seeming to acknowledge that I was making sense. Then, she would immediately shift back to wanting to know specifics about how to change her exercise routine or diet to get to where she was determined to go.

When she left I felt confused and defeated. This lovely and obviously bright young woman was going to continue on course, punishing herself for no good reason, avoiding self acceptance at all costs.

In follow-up sessions with Molly many months later, I learned that she had accomplished her goal and had reached her target weight. I also learned how she had almost killed herself to get there. She had taken laxatives by the box and medications to help her vomit everything she ate. She tortured herself to get off the hated 30 pounds. And when she got down to 150 pounds she was delighted and felt that she had finally arrived. Even so, she told me how she had nearly died; how horrible she felt physically; how she had undergone all sorts of tests in the hospital which revealed all manner of internal dysfunction. Still, the triumph of reaching 150 pounds superseded all this damage.

Eventually, her body went on a rampage and weight came back on quickly. This is when she came to see me. She didn't know what she weighed, as she was too afraid to step on a scale. We talked and I again reinforced everything I had told her before. She nodded again, but from little things she said it was clear that she longed to be back at 150 pounds and was prepared to sacrifice everything to get there again.

I wish there were a happy ending to this story. Maybe someday there will be. But for now Molly is still lost in her negativity and is still battling ferociously against her body.

To be sure, Molly's story is extreme. But the theme is widespread and common among American women.

3. THE DOUBLE STANDARD

The stories of Molly and Sarah and many similar experiences caused me to reflect on how I, as a man, have contributed to the thinness-at-all-costs insanity. Men, in general, are less nurturing, less caring, less supportive, less understanding, less empathic than women. We men are especially less so when it comes to women and their bodies.

Fred and Sue

Fred had a huge pot belly, but didn't see that he had a weight problem. On the contrary, his huge belly was solid as a rock, which to him meant that his protruding gut wasn't fat, it was simply the way he was built. He was comfortable with himself. But not comfortable with Sue, his wife. "She jiggles when she walks," Fred said. "She needs to firm up and get rid of that cellulite on her thighs."

I studied Fred and Sue. Fred had a weight problem. Sue did not. But, ironically, Sue agreed with Fred's assessment that she was unacceptable and that's why they sought my advice. They wanted a diet and exercise program for Sue—to cure her "jiggling." I wanted to smack Fred and bring him out of his fantasy world, and at the same time let Sue off the hook. But Fred and Sue were co-conspirators here; both were responsible for their distorted view of reality, both assumed that Sue needed fixing, while Fred was doing just fine.

Fred's giant belly was hard as a rock because the fat around his middle was stored below the abdominal muscles, pushing the muscles outward, stretching them like banjo strings. This is typical of male pattern fat storage. Sue, on the other hand, tended to store much of her fat just below the skin and on top of the muscles —subcutaneous fat storage. Thus, even a modest amount of concentrated subcutaneous fat resulted in a "waffled" appearance called cellulite, causing the thighs to jiggle while walking. (I will provide more detail on cellulite in Part II, #6.) In total, Sue had much less fat than Fred, but what she had was more visible.

From a health perspective, Fred's belly was much more dangerous than Sue's thighs. Sue, in fact, could triple the size of her thighs and the health danger would still be less than Fred's belly fat. The reason is, belly fat is easily mobilized (dumped into the bloodstream), flowing into the liver where it is converted to cholesterol, elevating the amount of cholesterol floating in the bloodstream which can contribute to clogging of the arteries.

Belly fat also is a player in insulin resistance which can lead to Type II diabetes, elevated serum triglycerides and hypertension (high blood pressure), greatly increasing the risk of heart disease. Female body fat on the hips, thighs and buttocks, on the other hand, stays put and doesn't generally endanger health.

As I looked at Fred and Sue I thought, "What's wrong with this picture?" But by now the scenario was so familiar that I just sighed and began explaining the ins and outs of their situation. Fred didn't much like what I had to say. Sue seemed confused at first, but eventually she seemed to understand that they had been viewing the world of weight management from a cock-eyed perspective. If anything, they should be seeking my advice for Fred, not Sue. Fred had far too much excess fat on his body, and the way he wore his fat increased his health risk in a number of ways.

I credit Sue for not telling Fred "I told you so!" Despite being bombarded by Fred to lose weight and shape up, she didn't succumb to the same tactics in retaliation. Not at all. Instead, she was immediately concerned for Fred's health status. Perhaps both of them could benefit from a dramatic change in lifestyle, she suggested, continuing to support her stubborn husband. But Fred wasn't buying it. He knew fat when he saw it, and he could see the fat on Sue and that was the problem. I could tell by the look on Sue's face that this was a battle I wasn't going to win. I let it go and bid them farewell and good luck.

4. LESSONS FROM OPRAH

Oprah Winfrey is an icon. Everyone loves her, myself included. I'm a big fan not only of her TV personality, but also for her captivating humanness. Nowhere is her humanness more real or more relevant than in her struggles with weight. Oprah's story is every full-figured woman's story. The yo-yo ups and downs, the lack of confidence, self loathing, and in her words (from the book, *Make The Connection*, by Bob Greene and Oprah): "I felt so much like a loser, like I'd lost control of my life. And the weight was symbolic of how out of control I was. I was the fattest woman in the room." These were Oprah's thoughts the night she won the Daytime Emmy Award for Best Talk-Show Host. It should have been a time of celebration, a recognition that she was the best at what she does. Instead, her weight and the shame it brings denied her the joy of the moment.

Oprah's odyssey

Oprah's odyssey with weight is instructive in many ways. In 1976, at age 22, she copped the prize as co-anchor of a TV news program in Baltimore. She should have been on top of the world. But in reflection, she realized she was lonely and under mega-doses of stress trying to adapt to this new, highly charged and demanding situation. In response, she ate. Eating has a way of comforting, but it also packs on the weight and soon she weighed 148 pounds. In her words, "a whopping 148!" Panicked by her ballooning weight, she consulted a diet doctor and restricted herself to a paultry 800 calories a day. She dropped weight quickly by starving herself and soon was back to 140 pounds.

Did the weight stay off? Of course not. As I have preached for years, and have pounded away at in this book, you cannot lose fat quickly from your body. It's impossible, and that's a fact. Losing muscle and water is easy, however, and you can drop 10 pounds quickly. But you will gain it back just as fast. Your body will force you to, and indeed it did with Oprah, propelling her upward in no time to 150 pounds.

At 150, Oprah got serious about dieting. Like everyone else, she sought the magic bullet, going through diets, one after another, hoping to find something that would work and have a lasting effect. She recounts trying crazy diets which yo-yo'd her to 160 pounds, then 165. She tried every available weight loss program, went back to seeing the diet doctor, worked in groups with others desperate to lose weight. The result of her efforts over eight years? She weighed 172 pounds.

You'd think someone as bright and well-informed as Oprah would have awakened to the truth along the way. You'd think at some point she would have reasoned that all the things she was doing — all the goofy diets, all the programs — had certain common elements. And indeed they did. Starvation, deprivation, a sense of urgency, ridiculously high expectations, and, of course, the "fool-figured" mentality — an absurdly low target weight, one that did not fit her full-figured, real woman's body. Promises, promises, promises. Failure, failure, failure.

Then in 1983 came the big break and the move to Chicago. To her delight, Oprah discovered her weight was not an issue—the powers that be said she could weigh what she weighed, 172 pounds. But she found that living the high-life has a price, and that price was additional body fat. Soon she weighed 180. In her words, "I started feeling more self-conscious. Here I am, a whopping 180, and I was supposed to be losing weight to impress my new Chicago audience." After that, she zoomed up to 202, then more gradually to 218.

This called for extreme measures. Her next approach was a liquid starvation diet; she ate no solid food for four months. She was ecstatic, losing 11 pounds the first week, and 30 pounds in one month. Eventually, she got down to 142 pounds and back into her size 10 jeans. She was ready to share her story with the world, telling us how she did it. It made great news. It also inspired critics, professionals who knew exactly what she had done to herself (she had reduced her metabolism to a mere dribble —the effect heightened by losing lots of muscle; she hadn't used exercise as part of the regimen; she had lost the weight much too quickly; she hadn't learned any new lifestyle habits to help her sustain the weight loss, etc.). The critics warned that she would gain the weight back. Oprah swore she wouldn't.

Just two weeks after going public with her story, Oprah's weight zipped up to 155. One year later she was 168, then quickly 175. New resolve set in. New diet plans. More failure. More self loathing. Her weight crept upward to 196, then 203. At age 37 she was 226. Her self assessment at this weight: "So big, disproportionate, fat in the face." Her weight consumed her, capturing her thoughts every waking hour.

Then in 1991, Oprah had a bout of sanity. She vowed to quit dieting and to begin simply eating right, with nutritious low-fat foods. Her goal? To be healthy, despite her weight. It's not that she intended not to lose weight and to give up the effort entirely. Not at all. Losing weight was still in the back of her mind. The result? Despite hiring a chef to cook nothing but healthy foods, Oprah gained weight. Eating was her addiction, and eventually she reached 237 pounds — her weight when she stepped forward to accept her Daytime Emmy Award.

Bob Greene—personal trainer

Then Oprah met Bob Greene, a personal trainer. Bob is charismatic, inspirational, and well educated on the issues, and through long talks with Oprah he was able to explain to her why all her weight loss efforts had failed, how they could never have succeeded, no matter what, and why she *always* gained back the weight she lost. Bob, I'm pleased to say, emphasized many of the things I have advocated for years. He convinced her to quit weighing herself every day, to live a healthier lifestyle, and to develop the confidence that, given sufficient time, her body would make appropriate adjustments—adjustments that would last.

Oprah began working with Bob in early 1993. He got her walking, then jogging short distances, and eventually jogging three to five miles and competing in half-marathon road races. Ultimately, she hiked the Grand Canyon (carrying a heavy pack) and even ran a full marathon. By late 1993 she had reached her goal of 150 pounds. Oprah perceived herself as being "strong and lean and fit and healthy", and indeed she was. But it wasn't a smooth and stable journey. At times her weight jumped up by as much as 17 pounds. But she brought it back down and by the end of the book was staying, generally, in the low to mid 150's.

I wish this were the end of the story. But it's not. Oprah has gained weight again. Why? I don't know, but if Oprah is like others who have made this journey, I suspect it's because the lifestyle she had adopted under the guidance of her personal trainer was not authentic. It worked, of course, to produce a wondrous result. But her body, mind and soul, I suspect, believed she was living under false pretenses. The marathon running Oprah was someone else. That Oprah was living for the public, not for herself.

The lesson to be learned

What's to be learned from Oprah's 20-year odyssey? Something very important. In 1976 Oprah weighed 150 pounds. Was she satisfied at that weight? Obviously not. She perceived herself as fat and began destroying herself with one ill-fated weight loss scheme after another, each time losing weight quickly, then gaining it (and more) back just as quickly, all in pursuit of the mythical fool-figured look.

Why wasn't she satisfied? In her mind's eye, I suppose, she believed she needed to look like the sleek female stars of daytime soaps. Was this possible for someone with Oprah's genetic makeup? No. But the image was implanted deep in her psyche and it victimized her constantly, thrusting her through the gauntlet of weight loss hell.

But, you say, what about Oprah's good work with Bob Greene. Was that an ill-fated scheme? No. On the contrary, I have great admiration for what was accomplished. Bob Greene's method is great — scientifically sound, tried and proven. But the truth is, it didn't last. Why not? Oprah was forcing herself to sustain an unrealistic standard.

Oprah made a huge circle—150 pounds to 237 and back again with the help of Bob Greene. She stayed there for quite some time through superhuman effort, clinging, in effect, by her fingertips to the edge of a cliff. This tells you a lot about how determined she is, and the incredible stuff she's made of. But it was inevitable that, in time, she would let go. And she has. Does this mean she has failed? Not at all. It merely means she has victimized herself repeatedly with unrealistic expectations.

In my opinion, I respectfully offer that if Oprah's health

134

is not in danger, she should be allowed to weigh what she naturally should weigh. This would be somewhere in the middle of the extremes she has experienced. It certainly wouldn't be 237 pounds, nor would it be the unsustainable 150. Whatever it is, I encourage her to embrace herself as she is, in the same way all of us in this country embrace her. We could care less if she runs marathons and looks like a *Sports Illustrated* bathing suit babe. That's not Oprah!

But what if Oprah herself is not satisfied? So be it. She can make some changes, adopt my strategy and over the next few years shift gears and lose 10 pounds or 20 pounds per year, or less. This is accomplished by making subtle changes. Changes that aren't demanding, punishing, or extreme. Changes that are real, wholesome and intrinsic. And most important is the change in attitude toward self acceptance, rather than self loathing. In the process, Oprah can smile at her viewers in the TV audience, self-satisfied, confident, bursting with self-esteem, comfortable with her body, knowing we accept and love her just as she is.

If Oprah, and others like her in similar positions of great influence, can do such a thing it would be wonderfully liberating to the millions of women held captive by unrealistic expectations. It would be the rebirth of an older era, perhaps a return to the time of Lillian Russell, when women looked like real women and men loved every ounce of the female body.

Jane and Becca

Jane Brody, personal health columnist for *The New York Times*, writes in the foreword to the excellent book *Thin for Life* by Anne Fletcher (Houghton Mifflin, 1994): "People who have met me within the last 25 years find it hard to believe that I was once a third bigger than I am now." When the pounds began to mount, Jane dieted—"All kinds of diets." She'd lose weight only to have it reappear, "with some extra pounds to boot." Finally, she reached the limits of fatigue surrounding the foolishness of crash dieting and decided that she was destined to be fat and she needed to accept the fact. When she did she also decided that just because she was going to be fat didn't mean she had to be unhealthy.

In the pursuit of health she exercised uncommon sense and did some entirely sane things. She began working with her body, and quit working against it. She quit crash dieting, quit starving and bingeing, and started eating three healthy, nutritious meals a day. When the snack bug bit, she resorted to wholesome snacks, and occasionally, but only occasionally, she treated herself to old favorites—a bit of cake or pie, a cookie, or some ice cream. She also began an exercise program. Nothing special—no rocket science or high-tech stuff—just walking, cycling, swimming, tennis, etc.

The results of her uncommon common sense approach? She lost weight and has kept it off for 25 years. In addition, she improved her health and, just as important, she is satisfied, finally, with her body. Jane Brody lives exactly what I am recommending in this book.

Becca, my colleague at the Health Promotion Center, is another example. As a middle-aged woman, Becca had long since accepted the fact that she would carry an additional 20 pounds or so on her frame, and that she would never again have the body of a high school cheerleader. She felt okay about her body, in other words, and overall her attitude was sane and healthy.

When Becca came to work with me, her serum cholesterol was 265 mg/dl—a dangerously high concentration of cholesterol in her blood which could ultimately clog her arteries, possibly causing a heart attack (by far the leading cause of death in women). As a registered nurse, Becca understood the implications and we set out to overhaul her diet. Over a six month period during which she cut her saturated fat intake to nearly zero, she was able to drop her serum cholesterol concentration to 180. During that same time, however, she dropped 15 pounds of body fat. She did this without trying to lose weight. It simply happened because she was doing the right things to improve her health.

And lately, because of a newfound interest in dance, she exercises with dance groups several days a week and has lost additional pounds of fat. But all is not rosy for Becca. At times when her schedule becomes overwhelming the dancing goes out the window. So do the long walks. The result? A few pounds come back on. But she doesn't panic. She realizes her body is a dynamic entity, always changing, growing, shrinking, adapting to circumstances. The key is her sane approach to weight management. When times are bad, she knows her weight may increase, but she is confident there won't be a rush of additional pounds. Conversely, when times are good, the weight will come down again, slowly and surely.

Let me emphasize the importance of this go-with-the-flow easy approach to weight management which operates within reasonable boundaries. Ebbs and flows are natural and to be expected. But such ebbs and flows do not occur with crash dieting. On the contrary, typically, women crash off lots of weight, punishing themselves in the process. Then when the daunting task of sustaining their quick and excessive weight loss hits them, they are overwhelmed. They cannot imagine going through the rest of their life with such an uncomfortable lifestyle. Sure, for a while it was tolerable, because the weight was pouring off. But the quick weight loss was a distorted fantasy that couldn't be maintained. Knowing this, they quit. The weight rushes back on, and the whole business is an abject failure, destined to be repeated again and again.

The bottom line is, applying common sense, which, of course, is quite uncommon when it comes to weight management, is the only road to true success.

5. SHRINKING VIOLETS

As recently as one hundred years ago, actress Lillian Russell wowed the male public with her ample 200-pound figure, and audiences whooped and hollered in appreciation of this fleshy beauty. Today it's hard to imagine anything other than whoops and hollers of derision from a male audience for a 200-pound woman in a skimpy outfit. Then, a "real woman" was voluptuous and attractive. Today, a "real woman" is fat and ugly. What went wrong?

Obviously there has been a shift in our perception of what is ideal for the female physique. Question the average American, male or female, about how a woman is supposed to look and they'll point, perhaps, to a poster of a young Jane Fonda in leotards. We are taught at an early age that the ideal women is lean and willowy ("One can never be too rich, or too thin!") While the willowy look is the standard for today, it is substantially removed from what was once considered the ideal. A few hundred years ago the ideal woman was fleshy and round, rounder even than Lillian Russell. A visit to the nearest art museum will reveal just how round and fleshy women really were. Given today's standards, Rubens' models would be considered obese.

By today's standards, a woman of average height who weighs 160 pounds would be considered to have a "weight problem." All who know her would be convinced of it, and she, of course, would know it herself. Chances are good she would have a long history of dieting, her weight shooting up, tumbling down, shooting up again. But is her weight a problem? That depends. If we mean a "health problem," probably not. From all we've learned about obesity, the mere fact that her body carries extra flesh may not be a health problem at all.

But hasn't it been established that excess pounds contribute to major health problems, such as heart disease, stroke, cancer, diabetes and the like? Yes, but the evidence suggests that such problems may not be related to excess body fatness *until the degree of fatness reaches extreme proportions* in women. This means a woman of average height who weighs 160 pounds and who has health problems, may not be unhealthy because of her weight, but rather, because of her diet. Fix the diet and the health problems may go away, regardless of whether she loses body fat or not. (I'll discuss this in greater detail in Part II, #7.)

Health concerns are only one part of the issue. A major

aspect of a perceived "weight problem" is self image, which in our society usually translates to self loathing, diminished self esteem, and lack of confidence. Ironically, addressing health issues is much easier than correcting erroneous self perception. But that's precisely what we need to do. To get there, we must understand how American women have been hoodwinked into believing that being thin is the only way to go — the only way to be desirable, cool, sexy, and most of all, natural. Bunk! Being thin is about as natural as being morbidly obese. Both represent extremes. Extremes are best avoided.

Lillian Russell versus the Gibson Girls

The seeds of our current feminine despair can be traced to the early days of this century and a movement to improve the physical fitness of women. Health experts decreed that women need more exercise, but appropriate dress at the time with its multiple ballooning layers restricted physical activity and interfered with outdoor exercise. Clothing had to be changed to allow freedom of movement, and with the change came new ideas regarding ideal female lines.

The Lillian Russell look, with its voluptuous full-bosomed, hour-glass flow was abandoned in favor of the Gibson Girl look which emphasized a tight waist, but not one that was brought about by squeezing into a chain-mail corset. Women were expected to come by this look naturally. From that beginning, we progressed to the Flapper look with emphasis on a more boyish physique. Short skirts readily revealed critical review of the female anatomy, and anything other than a pencil-thin waistline, and wispy hips and thighs was taboo. The age of caloric restriction and dieting was upon us.

Another factor propelled the female obsession with weight to new heights. The power of the media flaunted its ideal of what a woman should look like and screen stars set the standard. From Theda Bara to Betty Grable to Marilyn Monroe, we gradually became less tolerant of excess flesh. In the 1950s Miss Americas had five foot six inch, 150-pound bodies. Today, Miss

America is several inches taller and forty pounds lighter.

In the 1960s, Twiggy epitomized the skinny look which took over as the ideal for magazine ads. Women yearned to wear the flamboyant and dramatic clothes they saw in these ads, but not until they had starved to the point where they could proudly display prominent collar and cheekbones. Even then, after losing more pounds than they should, women felt they still didn't measure up. Despite being obviously skinny (to the objective eye), they continued to see themselves in their mind's eye as too fat. They perceived themselves as frauds, pretending to be something they weren't. The era of the negative female body image had arrived.

Fat discrimination is alive and well

The story I told earlier about Molly (the young woman who lost 300 pounds but wasn't satisfied) is an example of how fat discrimination in our society can exert a profound impact on its victims. If you carry too much weight, you are viewed as lazy and self-indulgent. In the business world, this translates to being incompetent and a poor hiring risk. Sufferers are urged by friends and foes alike, supporters and detractors, to go on a diet. Get the weight off quickly and at all costs. Thin has now become synonymous with attractive. Thin is good. Fat is bad. The belief has permeated our society all the way down to our youngest children. Obese children are viewed with disdain and unworthy of friendship. So deep are these feelings, studies have shown that thin teens suffering from diabetes would not exchange their dangerous condition for obesity even though the health implications are considerably less.

Physicians, caretenders of our health, are guilty of the same bias toward their overweight patients, particularly women, spewing shame and humiliation on those who need their support and counsel the most. Many physicians believe their fat patients simply don't care. Fat patients are uncompliant and totally disinterested in their own well being, and as such, how can the doctor be expected to help those who won't help themselves?

Our society has become filled with double binds for the obese. Nancy Bryan tells us about double binds in her book *Thin is a State of Mind* (CompCare Publishers, 1980). She writes: "Gregory Bateson, who coined the term, defines a double-bind as a set of contradictory paths that punish you no matter which one you choose. A perfect example of a double-bind for an overweight female would be today's women's magazines, which feature alternating pages of luscious desserts and overly skinny models wearing the latest fashions. Eating as overweight people in our culture tend to do it is also a double-bind; at any given time most fat people are either dieting (in a spirit of self-pity) or bingeing (in a spirit of self-hate)."

It seems that almost every woman I know thinks she has a weight problem. Some perceive their problem as major, others view the problem with less zeal. Regardless, all view themselves as unacceptable the way they are. Indeed, fully 75 percent of American women think they are too fat. If they are not on a diet, they are thinking about starting a diet, or just finishing one. Some are thin, quite thin, in fact, and yet they cling to the belief they've got to take off another five pounds. And once the weight is off, they fret that they'll gain it back, which inspires the need to lose another five pounds as a security measure, just in case. This means, of course, that they can never be thin enough, and they will always have another five pounds to lose, no matter what. Is it surprising, then, that 11 million women are cursed with eating disorders?

The majority of women I know hate the way they look, and too many of them bounce back and forth between starving and stuffing themselves. Crash diets lead to the rapid loss of thirty pounds, followed by feeding frenzies which pack that thirty pounds and more right back on. Depression accompanies the diet, and after the diet there is deeper depression compounded by feelings of misery and failure and the further loss of self esteem as the weight is regained. How widespread is this problem? No one is certain, but polls suggest that at any given time as many as 30 million women are dieting to lose weight.

This fanaticism is not restricted to adult women. On the contrary, fully half of high school girls see themselves as overweight and more than two-thirds intend to lose weight. Girls as young as 6 to 9 years of age express distaste for those they believe are too fat, and girls as young as 5 and 6 years are concerned about the appearance of their bodies. Polls reveal that 3 million teenage girls regularly skip meals as a weight management tool and that most girls from menarche on desperately battle their fears of weight gain. As many as one in eight young women admit to being chronic dieters, and as many as one-third diet periodically as part of their "normal" lifestyle.

It's no wonder the weight loss industry is a highly successful multi-billion dollar enterprise. It's also amazing and ironic that the success of this industry is built upon expectations of failure. Women try one weight loss scheme after another, always searching in vain for the easy solution. Every month there is a new crash diet which promises instant weight loss. Check the shelves of any book store, and you will see diet books spanning several shelves. They proclaim the benefits of eating bizarre combinations of foods, loading up on fats and shunning carbohydrates, of drinking water by the gallon, of cutting calories to a subsistence level—the list goes on. And there are the gimmicks, the potions and lotions, the prescriptions and over-the-counter medications, hypnotic suggestions, and shock therapies. At the extreme we have invasive medical interventions which include stomach stapling, jaw wiring, liposuction and bowel bypass surgery.

Doris

In my dealings with women in recent years I have learned not to take anything for granted. Here's the story of Doris, a good friend.

Doris has a weight problem and at one point had lost nearly 90 pounds before hitting a plateau she maintained for nearly two years. She needed to lose another 90 pounds or so, but at least she hadn't digressed. Then she got enthusiastic again and began exercising in earnest every day; her weight again began to drop. In a matter of months the change in her was remarkable. She has a very pretty face, and the weight loss allowed her pretty features to again surface. But after a while she stopped her efforts. Doris suffers from bouts of depression and when she is depressed she "checks out" and goes deep inside, going through the motions of life but not living. Some weight came back, but she was still doing well.

A while later she got back on the wagon again. All in all, my view was that this ebb and flow was part of a natural process. When her weight fluctuated, it didn't zoom up or down. She had learned enough good habits from my tutoring to sustain her and not allow herself to be victimized too severely by periods of reduced effort. Overall, I was optimistic that she would get to a point where she was satisfied and would stay there. She would be "full-figured", in other words, and proud of it.

Then Doris met a man she liked and began dating. Chuck had a weight problem, weighing more than 400 pounds and had a basketful of health problems, including high blood pressure and diabetes—the kinds of problems you would expect from a sedentary, obese man nearing his sixties. Good, I thought. Doris will be a positive influence in his life and will turn him around, leading him away from the disastrous path he was following. And in so doing, Doris will be bolstered in her approach and resolve. Boy, was I wrong! Chuck had no interest in losing weight. Unlike Doris, the thought of losing weight, shaping up and improving his health and appearance never occurred to him. It was irrelevant to him — a man's man! Unfortunately, in no time, Chuck began to unravel all the good things Doris had been doing. Instead of Doris having a good influence on him, he was exerting a horrible influence on her. Her weight began coming back with a vengeance.

The story goes on, with bumps and turns. I share this story to make the point that I had underestimated Doris' lack of self confidence and lack of self esteem. She was dating after years of abstinence and didn't want to rock the boat, fearful that if she exerted herself she might lose her man. If it meant going along and destroying herself in the meantime, that was okay. Keeping the relationship alive was the most important thing.

In knowing the two parties involved, it is my belief that a bit of effort on Doris' part would most likely have been well received by Chuck. He may have tested her determination at first, but I believe he would have yielded and accepted her leadership and would have been much better off for it. But that was not in the cards. I suspect the root of the problem is that Doris was thankful for having Chuck in her life, believing at some deep level that because of her weight problem, she was undeserving, and damned lucky to have him—to have anyone. It wouldn't occur to her to apply that same reasoning to Chuck. He was extremely fortunate to find a woman like Doris to take him, given all of his foibles. But our society imposes such thinking in huge doses on women, leaving men off the hook.

Men are fat, too, but...

While this section is directed toward women, I am aware that fear and loathing of fatness is not entirely a female issue. But the role it plays in the female life is likely to be more profound. Ask Doris. Ask Chuck. Women are much more likely to obsess about their weight, go on a diet, and go out of their way to select clothes which mask their condition. Women, and especially young women, are more prone to eating disorders such as anorexia and bulimia. Men in our society can overcome shortcomings thrust upon them by their weight by being successful, by achieving high incomes and powerful positions.

Women, on the other hand, tend (traditionally) to view their path to success as being driven by their attractiveness, which helps them gain access to resources controlled by men. Being fat means being unattractive, which means women who are overweight are fated to go through life lacking success. A fat man can compensate by having a good-looking women hanging on his arm. An overweight woman, on the other hand, is afforded no such compensation from dating an attractive man.

All in all, when it comes to body weight, the deck is stacked against women in our society. A change in attitude is needed, of course, but changing society's attitudes is a major undertaking and it is important to understand the dynamics involved.

Arthur Schopenhauer (1788-1860), the German philosopher, taught us that new ideas are at first rejected, then ridiculed, then, finally, accepted as self evident. And so it is with social concepts. Clearly, my idea that we can return to the good old days—a time when women could proudly wear a few extra pounds—will be rejected out of hand by the masses, men and women alike. In fact, women may be the most outspoken critics because they have invested the most in the status quo. But eventually, as the appeal of such a notion takes hold, we will reach the stage where there is debate and controversy. After that, if a significant number of us believe this is the right way to go, our society will embrace the notion. Fortunately, such a flip-flop in values does not require the majority of us to jump on board. On the contrary, a much smaller proportion of our society can sway the issue, and after a time it will be not only acceptable, but expected, and the validity of the notion will become self-evident to all.

The bottom line is, social movements are likely to begin as absurd ideas. But if the ideas are logical and appeal to common sense, then the possibility that they will become mainstream is strengthened immeasurably. It only takes a spark to get a fire going.

6. FEMALE FAT CAN BE SO STUBBORN

When you stand naked in front of a full-length mirror, what do you see? If you are a typical adult American you see an excess of fat peeking at you from various parts of the body. The exact location of that excess fat is important for two reasons. First, it may determine the degree of health risk associated with

145

carrying excess body fat. Second, the location may dictate how easily that fat will come off.

When you wear a lot of fat around your waist, you take on the shape of an apple. This is called male pattern (also android, or abdominal pattern) obesity. Females tend to store fat on the hips, thighs and buttocks, giving them more of a pear shape. This female pattern is also called gynoid, or gluteal-femoral pattern obesity. The apple shape is not necessarily restricted to men, although it is most prevalent in males. Similarly, the pear shape is not restricted to women.

Fat is stored in two primary ways—deep in the body cavities (Fred's pot belly), and directly beneath the skin (in subcutaneous fat—Sue's jiggly thighs). Female pattern obesity emphasizes subcutaneous fat, resulting in jiggly thighs and unsympathetic comments from males. But most men have little room to boast, and good reason to keep quiet. Male pattern obesity emphasizes deep fat storage, which accumulates and pushes against the abdominal muscles, stretching them taut. This causes many men to assume incorrectly that because their protruding pot bellies are hard, they are not fat. This is a very wrong assumption, and should be pointed out the next time an unwelcome comment surfaces about flabby female thighs.

Enzymes control the action

Where fat is stored says a lot about how easily it can be burned off. Throughout the body, fat is stored in fat cells which comprise adipose tissue, a type of connective tissue. Dietary fat is stored in adipose cells with the aid of enzymes (lipogenic enzymes—the "in" enzymes). Enzymes also play a role in calling fat from storage (lipolytic enzymes—the "out" enzymes). Enzyme activity differs in various locations of the body, and this difference creates both good news and bad news.

Lipolytic ("out") enzymes in the abdominal area are highly active and can call large amounts of abdominal fat from storage and into the blood stream. This means that given an appropriate low-fat and low-sugar diet and a regimen of daily physical activity, abdominal fat can be reduced rather efficiently. This is attractive from a fat-loss perspective.

But there is a down side to abdominal obesity. When under stress, fat release is triggered by stress hormones, which increases the risk of heart disease. This is because when fat is dumped into the bloodstream in large amounts (and not burned off in exercise), it increases the body's production of cholesterol. There's more to the story. Abdominal fat cells tend to be larger than those found elsewhere in the body, and these large fat cells are associated with insulin resistance, increasing the release of insulin and the risk of maturity onset (Type II) diabetes. And since excess insulin can cause increased reabsorption of sodium by the kidneys and other bad effects, there may be an increase in blood pressure.

Good news / bad news

Fat stored on the hips, thighs and buttocks also is a good news/bad news situation. The good news is, you can store a lot more fat below the waist (40-60 pounds) without greatly increasing the risk of heart disease. This is true for both men and women. The bad news is, the lipolytic ("out") enzymes which call fat from storage are lazy in areas below the waist, and once fat is deposited in these areas, it's very difficult to remove. Fat that is deposited on the hips thighs and buttocks is zealously guarded by the female body. Fat in these areas is thought to have been deposited for a special purpose—providing life-saving nourishment for the newborn.

In ancient times when food was scarce and unpredictable, Mother Nature had to be certain there would be adequate sustenance for new babies. Unfortunately, she chose mom's hips, thighs and buttocks as storage sites, and she surrounded these areas with what at times seems like an impenetrable force-field. It is not uncommon for women to go to great lengths in an attempt to lose lower-body fat. I have seen women take up marathon running, which resulted in the loss of many pounds of body fat. Their faces become gaunt, their arms pencil-thin, their waistlines shrink to less than 20 inches around. But despite all this effort, the fat on the hips and thighs—the main reason for taking up running in the first place—is still pretty much intact.

So is it hopeless?

No. As most women lose sufficient body fat, progressively more and more will come from the lower body. But not at first. One reason may be that the body instinctively reduces fat stores which impact health, and we know that fat around the waist presents a health problem. Thus, the body may overreact, taking off upper body fat to the extreme, before shifting gears. Unfortunately, because most women do not stay on body fat reduction programs long enough to see the loss of lower body fat, they conclude that it's hopeless. It's not. My suggested approach eventually will make an impact on the lower body fat of most women. We have seen successes. You must accept, however, that you may not progress to your desired goal—the slim, trim, 18-year-old cover-girl look—no matter how hard you try.

Mother Nature also offers a window of opportunity that should not be overlooked. Recent research suggests that during breast-feeding after pregnancy, fat deposits on the hips, thighs and buttocks are vulnerable to reduction. The factors that guard this fat are temporarily removed, and fat from these areas can be more easily mobilized and used as fuel to support the newborn. Unfortunately, this opportunity arises when mom has more important things on her mind than exercising or eating smarter to reduce the size of her thighs. Mom has to concentrate on being mom, and in so doing, she misses the brief window of opportunity that has been opened to her.

Six months to a year after childbirth, mom succumbs to the urge to get back in shape. But by then, her body may be undergoing change again, back to her former state. All is not lost, however. It just might take longer.

I am aware that losing lower body fat can be frustrating and can cause you to take foolish steps. One such step is the purchase of costly creams and lotions. The other is investment in fancy exercise equipment which guarantees fat loss in specific areas. Sorry. Such quick fixes don't work.

Failure to lose weight in specific areas through natural means is one reason why surgical liposuction techniques have become so popular. Liposuction is the "vacuuming out" of fat cells. It's a radical approach, but obviously one with lots of appeal, because plastic surgeons who perform liposuctions are doing a lot of business. But this procedure is costly and not without risk, and even with excellent results, major changes are not possible.

It's only fair to add that men seek out liposuction, too. Their problem is "love handles"—those slabs of fat above the hips that hang over the belt. Love handles can bring tears to the eyes of even the most determined men. Why are love handles so stubborn? We know it's not because the fat there is being protected to provide energy to a newborn. Why then? No one is certain. But love handles appear to be an early site of fat deposition, and it's possible that the body employs a "first in/last out" scheme.

Cellulite

In addition to liposuction, a variety of quick-fix schemes have popped up, and you need to be aware that they absolutely cannot work. You must accept this in order to protect yourself from being taken in. Nowhere are such schemes more prevalent than in the treatment of cellulite. Say the word and images of waffled thighs and rippled "cottage cheese" butts appear. Say the word and drive women to tears, then to the drugstore in search of the latest lotions and potions. Billions have been spent in the vain attempt to rid bodies of this fiend.

Why would the Creator curse us with such a mean-spirited and persistent foe? She didn't. So-called cellulite is no different from other fat deposits. It's stubborn, because it usually is found on the hips, thighs and buttocks. Beyond that, it's just plain old fat that looks different. Here's why.

Your body stores fat in adipose tissue which is composed of crescent-shaped connective tissue cells called fat cells. Fat cells have a tremendous storage capacity, and when they are full, they look like blown-up hot-water bottles.

If we could peek beneath the skin at a fat pad, we would see a criss-crossing matrix of connective-tissue strands that form compartments similar to those of honeycomb in a beehive. When the fat cells that fill each compartment expand, the compartments swell, pressing against each other and forcing an outward bulge that pushes toward the skin. When this occurs, several factors will determine whether you develop the unsightly waffled look.

Women are more susceptible to the cellulite look than men because women store more of their fat just beneath the skin, whereas men store more of their fat as deep fat in the abdominal cavity below the muscles. The more fat you have just beneath the skin, the more likely bulges will show.

Even when men have a large stockpile of fat beneath the skin, they will often escape the rippled look. This is because the outer layers of a woman's skin typically are thinner than those of men, showing the contents underneath more clearly. Also, the connective tissue compartments (of the beehive) may be tighter and more restrictive in women and that increases the tendency of fat cells to bulge outward to a greater degree.

The effects of these factors are exaggerated in women because women concentrate their fat storage in the hips, thighs and buttocks. If fat stores were more evenly distributed around the body, the bulging rippled effect would be reduced substantially.

The concept of cellulite being a "different animal" was promoted by women's magazines and those who wanted to sell salves, creams and other bogus items to help get rid of this problem. Cellulite looks different, and because it shows up on the hips, thighs and buttocks, it's very difficult to lose. But cellulite is not different from fat elsewhere on your body, and it doesn't require special interventions.

Patience and persistence are required, as is an understanding that you can only take your body so far. Do the right things and let nature take its course. Obsessing about your hips and thighs will only inspire you to do desperate things. You've been there and done that, so why repeat a foolhardy act?

7. HEALTHY FAT — AN OXYMORON?

As if all the psychological and perceptual complications I've discussed were not enough, society has placed one more heavy burden on the obese. If you are fat, your health is in danger. Many medical experts tell us that obesity kills, insisting that as little as 10 pounds in excess of limits set by standard height-weight tables destroys health. Obviously, this emphasis on the negative health consequences of excess weight helps increase anxiety to the breakpoint.

It's time for the truth—about the politics of being thin, and the misconceptions surrounding the connection between weight and health. Making the connection is easy, dispelling it is more difficult. Let's start with how the connection came about and why it's held with such tenacity:

Fact: Americans, in general, are overweight.
Fact: Americans, in general, are, despite the best health care system the world has ever known, essentially an unhealthy group.
Fact: Americans who are overweight have a higher death rate.

Put these three facts together—bingo! There appears to be a relationship; and, of course, there is.

A look behind the scenes

A look behind the scenes questions the strength of this relationship. Consider that higher death rates may be due to the fact that older people have a greater risk of dying, and as we age we get fatter. It's the age, rather than the increased weight that spurs the increased death rate. No one would doubt that the morbidly obese individual, someone who is more than 100 pounds in excess of their ideal weight, is unhealthy and at increased risk of heart disease, stroke, cancer, or diabetes. Wouldn't such individuals improve their health with the loss of 100 pounds of body fat? Of course they would. The relationship, then, associates age and extremes in body fatness with death rate and health status.

But what about the woman who, cosmetically, appears to be overweight by, say, 20 to 30 pounds or so? Is there a connection between those excess pounds and health? *If there is a connection, it is not a strong one.* A way of testing the strength is to have such women lose weight and watch for changes in their health status. Research studies have done this exact thing and have observed no real change in health status among women who have reduced their weight over a number of years.

But, you say, isn't it true that if I lose weight I can reduce my blood pressure, my serum cholesterol, my blood sugar? Why else would my doctor be on my case to get the pounds off? Yes, this is true. But let's take a closer look. Simply taking off pounds with some flim-flam crash diet does not necessarily improve your health. In fact, the opposite may occur. But taking off pounds *in the right way* should help. The right way means a slow reduction in body fatness by following a nutritious diet accompanied by increased daily physical activity. In both scenarios, pounds are lost but the result may be substantially different, which suggests that lost bodyweight may not drive the process, may not be required, and may not even be relevant.

Lifestyle, obesity and health

Your weight reflects your lifestyle. If you are carrying around too many pounds of fat on your body, chances are good you are not careful about your diet, and/or you are a couch potato. Your diet is loaded with fat, saturated fat in particular, and you probably consume too much simple sugar and salt. You follow the diet of a typical American, in other words. And as far as exercise is concerned, you probably invest a great deal of effort trying to avoid it.

This means you are fat because you follow a lousy lifestyle. It also means you are unhealthy because of your lifestyle. Your body fatness and your health status are outcomes—they are what you reap for your efforts; one does not necessarily cause the other.

In order to test this way of thinking, scientists have intervened, changing lifestyles, without changing body fatness. How? Encouraging overweight individuals to exercise, but have them consume enough calories along the way so as not to change their weight. What happens? They become healthier. The same is true for diet. Change the diet by reducing saturated fat intake as close to zero as possible and by reducing the intake of sugar. Along the way increase overall caloric intake and thus there won't necessarily be a substantial change in body fatness, but there will be improvement in health status. The message is clear. You can improve your health without losing weight.

Please understand this does not mean your weight is an unimportant consideration. On the contrary, it is important, especially if you tend to store excess body fat around the waist. Abdominal obesity can influence insulin resistance, and thus reducing fat from the middle can produce a dramatic change in your health status. But, for now, the message is, the amount you should weigh is much more individualized and much less stringent than the typical height/weight tables would have us believe. Just because you are 20 pounds in excess of what the height/weight table says you ought to be, doesn't mean you need to lose 20 pounds in order to improve your health. That 20 pounds, in fact, could easily be within an ideal range for you as an individual. Your ideal weight could range from 130 to 165 pounds for example, which means your health status is likely to be pretty much the same (assuming all factors such as diet, daily exercise, etc. remain constant) regardless of where you are in that range. Moreover, if much of that fat is housed below the waist, your range could be extended further.

Margin of error

What does all this mean? It tells us that you have a much greater margin of error in your bodyweight when it comes to health issues. It tells us that when figuring your ideal weight, you can be more forgiving of yourself, less punitive. It tells us to concentrate on the practices which contribute to good health;

eating properly, regular physical activity, and paying less attention to the numbers on the bathroom scale.

The key to this whole business is establishing a reasonable target weight for yourself. If I can convince you that a bit of extra flesh can be appealing and that it does not negatively impact your health, then perhaps you will allow yourself to rest at a weight that is comfortable and can easily be maintained. This, rather than struggling relentlessly in pursuit of a fool-figured, fantasized cover girl ideal that is forever beyond your reach—pursuing the impossible, making yourself miserable in the process, convincing yourself you are a loser and out of control.

The choice is clear. It's time to set the record straight. A fleshy body can be healthy and beautiful. In preparing for the work that lies ahead, the place to begin is with a reasonable body weight range that suits your needs and desires. Be open-minded and gentle on yourself. The possibilities for improving your quality of life are endless.

8. I HATE MY HIPS, MY THIGHS, MY STOMACH, MY ARMS

While working on this section, a magazine article caught my eye. It was about women's bodies and their perceptions of themselves. Along with the article were several pictures of women with bodies ranging in size from a two to a size 14. The captions under the pictures were interesting. The woman who was a size 14 was quoted as saying "I only look in the mirror once a day, so I can focus on what's inside." From this quote it would seem that this woman isn't exactly proud of her body, and that's probably true. Her quote suggests that in her mind she has come to grips with the fact that she doesn't measure up physically, and therefore her only option is to concentrate on her inner beauty.

I studied her picture. At 5' 11" she had a pretty face, shapely legs and looked pretty darned good in her clingy short dark green dress. I saw no reason why she wouldn't catch her share of admiring glances from gents as she walked down the street. I saw that in her, but obviously she didn't.

What about the size two woman? Surely, she must love her body. Right? Maybe not. Her quote set me back. At 5'5" and a size 2, she says: "I live by the motto... 'People don't notice what you don't notice.'" Good motto, of course, but what could it possibly have to do with someone with her proportions; someone our society deems as highly acceptable. What aspects of her size 2 figure should she "not notice?" I sure couldn't find any. Unfortunately, her quote implies that she does her share of body bashing, even though she'd have to look hard to notice things that she would choose not to notice.

I shook my head at the absurdity of it all. Women are so critical of their bodies that nothing is acceptable to them. No matter how good things are (size two, for example) there are flaws—deep shameful flaws—that scream out for attention and require a conscious effort to ignore. "I hate my hips, thighs, stomach and arms" is the mantra of the modern American woman. This concept, despite being based in unreality, is so firmly entrenched that it has created its own reality, its own rules of self perception and conduct, and, of course its own economy with a vast assortment of diet schemes, potions, lotions and exercise gadgets designed to create a new and better and acceptable you.

Mind/body games

The size 14 woman looks in the mirror only once a day. Why? Because she is so confident of her appearance that it requires only one assessment daily? Of course not. She looks only once, then tries to put what she sees out of her mind, because it is so depressing to her. What a shame, and so unnecessary. Clearly, the relationship between her mind and her body has been knocked way out of whack. The damage to her self esteem is obvious, and the impact on her daily life no doubt is considerable.

In the same magazine article there was a picture of a 5'8", size 10 woman. Her quote seemed out of place. She said: "I love my curves. My body is all mine and all natural." How refreshing.

155

What is it about this woman that allows her to accept a body that typically, in our society, would be deemed as substantially less than perfect. How can this size 10 woman love her body, when a size 2 woman clearly has less than a love affair with hers?

Much of the answer is perception and attitude. In today's world, perception is reality. What we perceive is real. If I perceive that people like me, it's real to me, and it will influence my attitude. The reality of this perception will gain momentum and strength, because my attitude will inspire me to be confident, outgoing, friendly and eager to interact—all factors that will increase my likability. Conversely, if I believe I am unpopular, I will lack confidence, be withdrawn and avoid interaction. I will be viewed as aloof and unfriendly, and therefore unlikable.

Can you change your self perception and your attitude? Yes. Hundreds of self-help gurus have tried to get us to do just that for decades. Books like *The Power of Positive Thinking* tell us that what we think influences how we feel and what we do. You can think positive thoughts and become a positive person.

But, you say, it can't be that easy. On the contrary, it is. But you have to believe it, and that's the Catch 22. If you don't believe it, it won't work for you. In addition, you must approach your mind/body reprogramming mindfully. If you are not mindful of what you are doing, your efforts will fail miserably. Ask anyone who has gone this route and chances are good they will tell you they littered their home with positive self help slogans, played taped positive messages on the drive to work, and recited positive sayings in the mirror until they were blue in the face, but nothing happened. Why?

They knew nothing would happen and they merely played it out to show they were right. Unless you are fully committed and unless you are very careful about what you are doing, your mind will attach a little tag to every positive slogan or message. "I love my body," you repeat over and over out loud as you peer in the mirror, and your mind tags on at the end of each saying, "Not really, because my body is ugly." Such a haphazard approach, unfortunately, can make matters worse.

If you are not mindful about your approach, you will (as in the example above) encounter a battle between your outward expressions and your inner thoughts. Your outward expressions are trying to influence your subconscious mind, but your thoughts are subverting the effort. Not only that, but because your inner thoughts in the beginning are so much more powerful than your mindless outward expressions, your subconscious mind will listen to your thoughts while ignoring the expressions, thus enforcing even more deeply the negativity you are trying to escape.

Now, please understand what I'm saying here. I'm not saying that initially you have to believe the positive slogans. That's asking too much and it's not reasonable to assert that you will be able to set aside years of negativity and immediately start believing that you are beautiful and acceptable just the way you are. Instead, what I'm saying is that you must believe that the process of bombarding yourself with positive messages works and will eventually pay off with a change in attitude. You must, in other words, believe in the process without focusing all your attention on the words.

Ten things to consider

1. **Use positive affirmations**. Seems stupid, I know, to tell yourself you are beautiful, when you clearly don't believe it. That's okay. You are not trying to reason with or convince your conscious mind. If that were your intention, you'd be wasting your time. You are instead trying to reach your subconscious mind and convince it. The good news is that if you put enough effort into it, you *will* convince it, and when you do the impact will eventually percolate to the surface and you will begin to believe what your subconscious mind is telling you. It's like a big circle. You reprogram your subconscious mind so that ultimately it can reprogram you. It's much like working with computers. It's important to program your computer correctly so that when you need it to give you something back, you have confidence that it is giving you what you need.

2. Add power to your affirmations by speaking them out loud to yourself (You don't have to do it when others are around). When you speak out loud, you focus more acutely and more forcefully and your subconscious mind tends to listen with greater attention and soak in what you have to say. It will feel a little strange at first, but hang with it because there is much to be gained.

3. Choose your affirmations carefully. There are many books filled with wonderful affirmations. You can scan such books and pick out the ones that you like and that you think will work for you. Or you can create your own. Regardless of your preference for personal or scripted affirmations, use them vigorously. They are powerful tools. Not only will they help reprogram you, they may influence your entire universe.

4. Be on guard against negative thoughts. You won't be able to eradicate them from your mind, but you can learn to spot them and kill them before they grow. Essentially, you are engaging in a healing process, and the rules of healing are pretty straightforward. Once you have removed the impediments to healing, healing will occur. The doctor does not heal your body, for example, you do. The doctor's job is to create the best set of circumstances possible for healing to occur.

Similarly, when "healing" your thoughts you must remove the impediments to creating the best set of circumstances possible. The impediments are negative thoughts and feelings. When these are removed, a positive healing process will occur naturally. You will gravitate toward the positive as if it were a great magnet, because that is where you naturally want to be.

5. Be thankful. I don't care how bad things seem, there are always things to be thankful for. Your health, your job, your parents, your children, your home, your car, the shade tree in your yard, the rain, whatever. Being thankful is one of the most powerful ways of being positive. How can you be negative when you are being thankful? You can't!

6. **Elevate your personal status.** Whose opinion of you is the most important? The answer should be obvious. It's *your* opinion of you that is most important. An old analogy applies here: If I died tonight, how many people would be upset to the point of tears? A few, to be sure, and of those few, how often would they think of me? If they are normal and involved in their own lives, the answer is... not often. A fleeting thought perhaps. So if all you are getting is a fleeting thought, why burden yourself with so much effort trying to measure up to what you think their expectations are of you, and seeking their approval? Chances are good that you already have their approval. And if they don't care about you, what difference does it make? That gets us back to the person who cares most about you—you. Your opinion of you is the most important. Elevate your opinion of yourself and in the process elevate yourself.

7. **Become a student of your pursuits.** The more you know, the more effective you will be. Study and learn not only what to do, but why you are doing it and why it is the right thing to do. Learn the lessons taught in this book and build on them. It may, for example, be difficult to swallow that you are doing much better in the weight management department than you thought. Years of telling yourself you are too fat and unacceptable are not easy to overcome. You will overcome, of course, and a good way is to learn as much as you can about the issues. You now know that our society's view of what a woman's body should look like has changed over the years. Take time to do a little historical checking on your own and study this issue. Take a look at what's going on in other cultures to broaden your view even further. This approach will help place things in meaningful perspective and will help you accept them more easily.

8. **Know that you can change some things about yourself and take steps to do just that.** The Serenity Prayer is particularly

applicable here. It asks for strength to change the things you can, strength to accept the things you cannot change, and the wisdom to know the difference between the two. Yes, you can improve your health by changing your lifestyle. Yes, you can alter your physique somewhat. But, no, you probably cannot get your figure back to the way it looked at the age of 17, before giving birth to two children and 25 years of living took its toll. You probably will never again have the hips, thighs, stomach and arms of a young girl. Accept this as a fact of life and quit swimming so hard against the current, trying to be something you cannot be. Such effort is punishing and self-defeating and makes life hard to live. Living is the most important thing we as human beings can do. Start now!

9. **Be gentle on yourself.** Fill yourself with praise for even the simplest accomplishment. Affirm yourself at every opportunity. Gradually move through the gauntlet of self growth, away from self loathing, to self acceptance, and ultimately, to self love.

10. Above all, **know that love is the most powerful force there is.** Harness it and use it to your advantage. Work with your body in love; quit working against it in fear. Your body will thank you and will reward you.